PRAISE FOR *THE METAB(*

"Tried everything you can think of to lose weig[...]er; it's your liver. You'll discover how to detox you[...] *sm Reset Diet*."

—JJ Virgin, CNS, *New York Times* bestselling author

"Dr. Christianson is my go-to expert when it comes to healthy liver function and natural weight loss. *The Metabolism Reset Diet* will empower you to take back your health!"

—Dr. Izabella Wentz, *New York Times* bestselling author of *Hashimoto's Protocol*

"We live in an increasingly toxic world and our livers are carrying the burden. Dr. Christianson's groundbreaking work reveals the missing ingredient we've been overlooking. If you're tired of diets and programs that have failed you, it's time to hit reset. I highly recommend this book."

—Dr. Pedram Shojai, *New York Times* bestselling author of *The Urban Monk*

"I love that *The Metabolism Reset Diet* cuts through the stress of fighting with carbs, fats, and ketones and delivers a way to eat simple healthy foods and not worry anymore. In a detailed and easy-to-understand way, this book explains how the liver holds the key to our metabolism and how to optimize it for life."

—Katie Wells, founder of WellnessMama online and author of *The Wellness Mama Cookbook*

"If you want an easy-to-follow, proven plan to lose weight and keep it off, and to improve your health for decades to come, you absolutely need to read this highly recommended book! In *The Metabolism Reset Diet*, Dr. Christianson does a superb job to shatter outdated myths related to weight loss and dieting. You don't need a restrictive food plan. You don't need to spend hours at the gym. The ingredients for sustained weight loss and to turn back the clock on aging are here."

—Steven Masley, MD, FAHA, FACN, FAAFP, CNS, author *The Better Brain Solution*

"Dr. Christianson has done it again—he's broken the mold on the carb, ketone, and fat conversation with an easy-to-follow program that relies on the solid science of metabolism and the ancient wisdom of food as medicine. If you're frustrated because you've tried everything, I believe you're in for a pleasant surprise that will wake up your liver's innate healing capacities and move you toward the optimum health you deserve."

—Aviva Romm, MD, author of *The Adrenal Thyroid Revolution* and director of the Women's Integrative Medicine Institute

the metabolism reset diet

Repair Your Liver, Stop Storing Fat,
and Lose Weight Naturally

By Alan Christianson, NMD

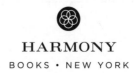

HARMONY

BOOKS · NEW YORK

The material in this book is for informational purposes only and is not intended as a substitute for the advice and care of your physician. As with all new diet and nutrition regimens, the program described in this book should be followed only after first consulting with your physician to make sure it is appropriate to your individual circumstances. The author and publisher expressly disclaim responsibility for any adverse effects that may result from the use or application of the information contained in this book.

Copyright © 2019 by Alan Christianson, NMD

All rights reserved.
Published in the United States by Harmony Books, an imprint of Random House, a division of Penguin Random House LLC, New York.
crownpublishing.com

Harmony Books is a registered trademark, and the Circle colophon is a trademark of Penguin Random House LLC.

Originally published in hardcover in the United States by Harmony Books, an imprint of Random House, a division of Penguin Random House LLC, New York, in 2019.

Library of Congress Cataloging-in-Publication Data
Names: Christianson, Alan, author.
Title: The metabolism reset diet / Alan Christianson, NMD.
Description: First edition. | New York: Harmony Books, [2019] | Includes index.
Identifiers: LCCN 2018030158 | ISBN 9780525573463 (pbk.) | ISBN 9780525573456 (ebook) diets—Recipes.
Classification: LCC RM222.2 .C484 2019 | DDC 613.2/5—dc23
LC record available at https://lccn.loc.gov/2018030158

ISBN 978-0-525-57346-3
Ebook ISBN 978-0-525-57345-6

PRINTED IN THE UNITED STATES OF AMERICA

Book design by Andrea Lau

10 9 8 7 6 5 4 3 2 1

First Paperback Edition

To Kirin Christianson, for being my biggest fan, loudest cheerleader, and most helpful critic for more than twenty years. Thanks, honey, I love you.

contents

the metabolism reset diet

THE METABOLISM MYSTERY

Maybe you've glanced at the plate of a coworker or friend and thought: Why can she indulge in that second piece of birthday cake—without tracking it or logging hours at the gym or feeling guilty for days—and stay naturally slim while I limit myself to a forkful and feel constantly fatigued and deprived and plagued with cravings . . . and overweight? Is there something wrong with me?

Here's the essential truth that I hope will propel you into a new chapter of thinking about yourself and your health and your weight: There is nothing wrong with you.

Naturally thin people are not superior. They don't try harder, nor do they possess superhuman willpower. They don't have better genes, and most don't eat fewer calories. They simply have one thing working in their favor: they have a better metabolism.

But for now, let's take assessments of "good" or "bad" out of it. The word *metabolism* is thrown around a lot in relation to diet and weight loss, but what does it actually mean? Your metabolism is simply how you convert fuel into energy. Fuel comes in as food. You never get exactly the right amount of food on a given day, but when you have a healthy metabolism, you can store a little extra food without gaining weight. That second piece of birthday cake isn't going to make or break you. You can also miss a meal without your energy levels crashing.

When the metabolism is not working properly, we store too much fuel and we are unable to retrieve it. This leads to extra pounds and a host of other adverse effects—everything from brain fog to digestive problems to fatigue to diabetes to various forms of cancer.

There's a common misconception that you are born with either a great metabolism or a bad one. But turns out that metabolism is not fixed. You can change. The key to this change is not in white knuckling it while the rest of your friends and family enjoy their lives, nor is it in forever eliminating your favorite foods. The secret that I discovered in my years of clinical practice and research is simply this: Clean out your liver so that it can burn fat better.

IT'S ALL ABOUT YOUR LIVER

The liver probably isn't even in the top five body parts you consider when you think weight loss, but it should be. The liver is more than just an organ damaged by alcohol or a quivering dish you'd prefer to avoid. It's the heaviest internal organ and the largest gland in your body. It's a powerful machine that acts as a filter to remove toxins, aids in digestion, and regulates hormones and blood sugar. It's an incredible multitasker and a vital organ in the truest sense of the word—the hub through which your body's energy flows. The liver is responsible for processing everything you ingest, and it also functions as your body's storage pantry. Nutrients (vitamins, minerals, and other substances the liver needs to work at its best) and fuel (from our main calorie sources—fats and carbohydrates) you do not need today are stored in the pantry for later. The surplus is essential because you never get exactly what you need each day. If you miss a meal one day, you should be able to draw on your surplus to compensate. And if you overeat, you should be able to store the extra for use on those days when you may not have enough time to take a bite. A healthy liver stores extra energy and doles it out later when you need it.

What happens when your liver is unhealthy? You tend to store fuel as fat, especially around your midsection, and you can no longer tap into the nutrients you need to burn fat. This means that no matter which diet you choose—and how hard you try—weight loss is pretty much impossible.

Sound familiar?

Countless diets have told us to eat this "good food" and avoid that "bad food." Meat, grains, butter, legumes, ketones, potatoes, tofu, canola oil—are they good or bad? Each passing day seems to bring a new wave of "science" that cancels out all previous assessments. In fact, fat, carbs, and ketones work collectively as fuel. A healthy liver can either store fuel or burn it. An unhealthy liver can only store it. All sources of fuel look the same to your liver—none are magic tonics or evil villains. This means that once you heal your liver, eating that piece of cake won't be catastrophic. Your metabolism will be flexible enough to adapt and handle whatever curveballs you throw its way.

That's very good news. And even better news? Healing your liver takes weeks—not months or years. The liver is an astonishingly resilient organ. With the steps I'm going to give you in this book, you can restore it to perfect working order in just a few weeks.

WHY THIS MATTERS TO ME

When people meet me, many assume that I am naturally thin. I take it as a compliment, but in fact when I was young I struggled with my weight. I was born with cerebral palsy and epilepsy. Perhaps being unable to be physically active put me at risk for weight gain. The first time I was obese was when I was eleven years old. Overweight kids were over three times rarer in the 1970s than they are today, so I stood out.[1] Fat discrimination and fat-shaming are still injustices these days, but back then they were not even concepts; they were just the normal state of affairs. What is now often still held as a private belief was then publicly shared—it was assumed that anyone who was overweight just needed to try harder.

In fact, I was anything but lazy and I tried hard at everything I put my mind to. I hated how I looked and I wanted to change. Willpower was not the problem. Besides my weight, it seemed that I could push through any obstacle. I knew that I had no less persistence than my thin peers did.

I went to the doctor, but his solution of logging calories didn't work. It wasn't until I turned to health books that I was able to make a difference. I read everything I could get my hands on, and based on the advice I gleaned, I cut out sugar, butter, and bread completely. I didn't touch any of those three foods for about a decade. My parents indulged a family member who sold multilevel supplements. Thankfully, this meant that we had protein powder available, and I started every day with a protein shake. For lunch and dinner my mom made good meals with whole foods. I added beginner exercise routines designed for sedentary people, and slowly but surely, I saw things change.

Once I got healthier, my life transformed. I felt better about myself, more confident and capable. For the first time, I came to experience the joy of movement. My physical abilities improved almost on a daily basis and I loved it.

In my mind, I owed my new lease on life to the health experts who shared their advice in books. They were my heroes, and I wanted to follow in their footsteps, so I decided to pursue medicine as my life's work. My transformation even guided my focus within medical school. I became fascinated by hormones because of their seemingly enigmatic role in regulating body weight. I knew how emotionally powerful my own struggle had been and how much effort it took. My heart went out for those in the same place who worked just as hard, yet saw no results. I dedicated my career to helping them.

While working with diabetics, I was exposed to the idea of modified fasting as a means to improve health. I read studies from 2011 in which advanced diabetics became cured by following a 600 calorie, liquid-only diet for eight weeks. The process sounded extreme, but so were the results. Blood tests and CT scans showed that these patients' pancreases had completely healed and were able to produce insulin normally. They no longer needed medication at all. It turned out that once their livers cleared out the old deposits of fat, they became nondiabetic.

This was a huge finding, and a surprising one as well. Historically we'd thought of the pancreas as the master organ related to diabetes—and once you were on a diabetic track, it was as if you were strapped to a runaway train. But this new research showed that the pancreas is only part of the picture. The liver also plays a crucial role because it has a remarkable ability to heal.

After reading all the related studies I could find, I asked several patients if they would be willing to try something new. My idea was that many who were pre-diabetic, or had less advanced diabetes, would be able to heal with a less intensive regime.

Instead of three liquid shakes, I tried two shakes and one reasonable meal. The results were tremendous. I tracked people every two weeks and saw that most achieved remission from diabetes well before eight weeks. The goal of the early program was diabetes reversal, and our clinic has logged countless cases of those who did just that. They became non-diabetic, stopped their medication, and continue to remain healthy years later.

Nearly everyone we treated had fatty liver syndrome, even though few ever had heard the term before. When the liver is overburdened by excess sugar, the body stores it as fat. This can trigger a potentially devastating inflammatory response, which has been linked to heart disease and some forms of cancer. What's more, new research suggests that fatty liver is not just *the consequence* of weight gain, it can also be *the cause* of weight gain. So addressing fatty liver syndrome is crucial in the fight to both regain health and lose inches. And the protocol I was sharing with my patients was working miracles.

Besides benefits to diabetes and liver function, the program cured a high percentage of people from high blood pressure, high cholesterol, and autoimmunity. I also noticed that as their liver function improved, weight loss happened naturally and came mostly from the waist. People were always happy to be free of disease, but they were ecstatic about the side benefit of weight loss. Many had inches that had lingered for decades—suddenly gone.

In our clinic, my team and I were so excited about the results that we all used the program ourselves for weight loss and learned how easy it was to stick with it. Next, we recommended it to patients who wanted help with losing some unwanted inches. They not only lost the inches, but reversed diabetes, lowered blood pressure, healed fatty liver, and ended autoimmunity. The results were so astounding that we began to recommend it as a solution for those conditions. Often it was the only step that people needed to regain their health.

My team and I became convinced of two points:

1. The program worked for people for whom countless diets failed them. They could lose weight for the first time and keep it off for years.

2. Weight loss of even a few pounds is the most surefire path to greater vitality.

THIS IS PERSONAL

The program you now have in this book follows the program that resulted in thousands of pounds of weight loss for participants. *Participants* is another word for people. People who have lost inches and reclaimed their health—and found a new lease on life just like I did as a young boy. I'm thinking of Shannon, a woman in her early 40s who'd developed thyroid disease. She'd put on 45 pounds, and she tried everything, including thyroid treatment, but the scale wouldn't budge. She felt constantly heavy, bloated, gassy, and uneasy. What's more, before she'd gained the weight, she loved participating in fitness competitions. Now not only was she unable to enjoy her favorite pastime, she didn't feel comfortable around her friends, most of whom she'd met in the fitness world. She felt an incredible sense of loss; she wanted to get back to her old self, her real self, but she couldn't figure out how and was starting to wonder if it would ever happen. I felt for her and I hoped we could help. She was one of the first people to participate in our clinical trials. She lost 14 pounds in the first four weeks, and I encouraged her to continue with the partial program. She cycled in and out of the program three or four times and ultimately lost all 45 pounds.

Imagine what that feels like. Imagine walking up a stairway with 45 pounds in a backpack strapped to you. Take off the backpack and suddenly it's as if you're walking on the moon. You feel like a new person. Shannon also had pre-diabetes and those symptoms were now completely gone. Being overweight and unhealthy can readily cut a person's lifespan short by a decade. So not only did Shannon have her life back now, she regained a decade in the future. Imagine what you could do with an extra decade—and a healthy, vital decade—how much time you could spend with your children or your friends and loved ones, all the things you could enjoy.

CLINICALLY PROVEN, ROAD-TESTED RESULTS

The program in this book is based on years of testing and refinement, with the helpful input of tens of thousands of participants in our clinical trials.

Between 2014 and 2016, I gathered statistics from participants in our clinic and those who followed the program online. The participants were mostly female, between the ages of 33 and 67 with a median age of 54. Some just wanted to lose a few pounds or an inch or two, some had goals of much more weight loss. The average goal was 3 inches and 23 pounds.

By the end of the four weeks, the average amount of weight loss was 13 pounds and the amount of "waist loss" was $2^{1}/_{2}$ inches! Most had reached their goal or were within a half inch of it.

Notice that they came closer to their waist goal than their weight goal. That was because they lost more weight from their midsection and little if any from their muscles, which is exactly what you want if you're looking for sustainable weight loss.

In the following months and years, I was able to reconnect with many of them. The typical theme was that immediately after the four-week reset, if they regained weight it was only a pound or two, but the inches did not seem to come back. They also talked about how they were no longer slaves to exact foods and exact portions. Their weight, energy, and appetite stayed on track even with the occasional unplanned meal or snack that life throws our way.

HOW IT WORKS

Your liver needs nutrients from your diet to help it get rid of the extra fuel it has accumulated. The Metabolism Reset Diet is carefully constructed to provide your liver the nutrients it needs without giving it more fuel to deal with. You'll achieve this goal with a 28-day program that offers healthy amounts of protein, fiber, micronutrients, and phytonutrients that support liver function. The program provides the right amount of fuel from carbohydrate and fat to prevent nutrient deficiencies while still prompting the liver to use its own supplies of stored fuel.

After just four weeks, you will be able to eat reasonably healthily and maintain your weight without any special effort. Most people find they can be less restrictive with food than they were before and still reap the benefits of a well-functioning liver. After liver function improves, people notice additional benefits like fewer food cravings, steady energy levels, less fluid retention, and better digestion.

Some will hit their weight goals in the four-week Reset, others will want to go further. If you finish your first Reset and still wish to lose more, the Metabolism Reset Diet includes a maintenance plan that provides foods that protect the liver from getting overloaded again. Those who complete the four weeks and wish to lose more weight can repeat a Reset up to once per three months—up to four times per year without slowing their metabolism.

You can also choose to make the Metabolism Reset Diet a yearly habit to assure your metabolism stays healthy and to stay vital for life.

The biggest benefit of the four-week program will be that you can regain metabolic flexibility and join the ranks of the naturally lean. The best part is that this change will not come about by avoiding "bad" foods or taking special supplements. Instead, it will come from an unclogged and healthy liver and its ability to manage your energy sources more carefully.

On finishing the book, you will be able to take control of your health and weight without having to follow a restrictive diet plan. I know the agony of living in a constant state of deprivation. I cannot wait for you to be free of the burden.

chapter one

Regaining Metabolic Flexibility

Belinda wanted to lose 17 pounds before her high school reunion. All her friends were talking about the latest craze, the ketogenic diet, so she decided to give it a try. For two months, she was religious about keeping her protein intake under 40 grams per day and her carbs under 20 grams. She did not worry about her intake of dietary fat, and stopped eating when she was no longer hungry. She followed the program to the letter, though she decided not to watch the scale since she did not want to be disheartened by normal ups and downs.

Near the end of the two months, Belinda saw her gynecologist for a well-woman check. When they weighed her, she was nervous, she was hopeful, and then she was heartbroken. She was 10 pounds heavier than before starting on the ketogenic program. She had seen the same thing happen on other diets but hoped that this time it would be different. When her blood tests came back, her gynecologist told her that she had an underactive thyroid and referred her to one of my colleagues at Integrative Health, Dr. Linda Khoshaba.

Dr. Khoshaba confirmed that Belinda's thyroid was underactive, and found that her metabolism was about half as fast as it should have been. This finding confirmed Belinda's experience—she was unable to lose weight no matter how hard she tried.

Belinda was encouraged when Dr. Khoshaba told her that her abnormal thyroid function was likely a side effect of her dieting—and that she could probably restore normal function by following the Metabolism Reset Diet and taking an iodine-free blend of nutrients to support her thyroid and liver. At first, Belinda was concerned because it looked like she would eat more food than she did on the ketogenic diet. But she gave it a try, and during the 28-day cycle, Belinda lost the pounds she gained during the ketogenic diet and then some. She was over the moon.

Three months after completing her first Reset, her thyroid and metabolism were both working fine. She was able to keep her weight steady without starving herself.

WHY DIETS HAVE FAILED YOU

Many of those who I saw in my clinical practice were like Belinda. They were driven, savvy people who had tried hard to lose weight. They'd given it their all on five or more diets in the last few years and experienced limited success. They typically saw things get better on the scale, but ended up with less metabolic flexibility than they began with and often found themselves back at square one—or sometimes even worse than square one.

When your liver isn't functioning properly, it is full of fuel but your body cannot use it. As a result, your body goes into a state of high stress and ends up using muscles as a source of fuel. If you are prone to depression or anxiety, stress makes it worse. Relationships suffer. In this state, are you motivated to exercise? No. Are you your best at work? Definitely not. On top of all the other physical and mental stress you're enduring, you also have to cope with intense cravings. Nearly every moment of the day you're fantasizing about your favorite foods rather than focusing on what really matters.

If somehow you managed to white knuckle it and stick with a major food restriction for months, maybe you could drop a few pounds. However, because your liver burns muscle rather than fat, you often end up lighter but with a slower metabolism. You weigh less (for now) but you also burn fewer calories. This means whatever weight you lost is likely to come back, even if you're still watching what you eat.

What shifted for Belinda is the same thing that will shift for you once you start this program. Your liver will regain its ability to manage your metabolism. Once that happens, your weight and energy will stay steady even though your diet may change. You will know what it feels like to be naturally thin.

Once you restore your liver function you'll be able to maintain a healthy weight without Herculean effort. And what's more, you'll have more energy, sleep better, and be at less risk for heart disease and many cancers.

I want you to succeed, and I believe that you can—even if you do not yet think it is possible. I have seen countless people do so even when they:

- Suffered from cravings
- Had myriad diets fail
- Were too busy to exercise
- Did not know how to cook

- Were overwhelmed with their family, their career, or both
- Had dietary restrictions
- Were on the road too much

The Metabolism Reset Diet works because it heals the core issue behind a slow metabolism—an overloaded liver. The program provides the perfect conditions to help the liver clear out its backlogged fuel and start working right again—and regain metabolic flexibility that you may not have experienced since you were a child.

WHAT IS METABOLIC FLEXIBILITY?

Our ancestors needed metabolic flexibility to survive. When food wasn't readily available, they could survive on what they'd stored for a time by breaking down fat to use as fuel. Most of us in this country live in the opposite type of environment: food is super-abundant. As a result of constant availability, we tend to overeat foods high in sugar, which causes us to store fat and impedes us from switching from one source of fuel to another. We become metabolically inflexible.

In order to see what this looks like in real life—and how it affects our lives and our waistlines—let's look at two examples.

Jane, a thin woman with a perfectly healthy liver, pays little attention to diet or exercise but does not need to—she has a great metabolism. One day, Jane finds some leftover muffins sitting out at work. Absentmindedly, she eats a few of them in addition to her normal diet. Her liver has room to store the extra fuel.

The next day, there are no muffins. Jane is so busy that she completely misses lunch. Her liver withdraws some of the fuel it had socked away from yesterday's muffins. It keeps her energized and alert despite her missed meal.

Jane has a flexible metabolism. Her liver is able to store fuel and withdraw it as needed. Even though she does not always eat the correct amount of food, her weight is steady and she feels fine.

Now let's consider Jeanette. She also had extra muffins one day and no lunch the next. Her liver didn't have room to store the extra fuel. So when she missed a meal and her body needed energy, her blood sugar levels dropped off and she crashed. This left her feeling mentally cloudy, tired, and edgy. She also had terrible sugar cravings later in the day because her body needed a quick source of fuel. So she gorged on ice cream the minute she got home and felt helpless against this cycle of cravings.

RESET TO THE RESCUE

At some point in our lives, nearly all of us had metabolic flexibility like Jane's. Maybe it was only in early childhood, but there likely was a time when you ate what you felt like and played as much as you wanted to. Despite a food intake that was not perfectly matched to your day's needs, your adipose levels were appropriate and your energy lasted throughout the day. You still got hungry, but hunger was not your enemy.

This is metabolic flexibility and it is your birthright. I'd like to help you get it back.

HOW FLEXIBLE IS YOUR METABOLISM?

Take this quiz to find out how flexible you are. Read the following questions. Place a mark in the "Yes" box if you feel that the question applies to you. Place a mark in the "No" box if it does not. Count the "Yes" marks to determine your score.

	QUESTION	YES	NO
1	I often get bad food cravings.		
2	I can gain 2 pounds or more overnight.		
3	I do not lose weight when I exercise hard.		
4	If I miss a meal, I feel edgy or exhausted.		
5	I often wake in the middle of the night.		
6	I would gain weight faster if I ate like my friends.		
7	I often feel bloated.		
8	I need coffee to get going in the morning.		
9	I often feel spacy or distracted.		
10	Eating sugar makes me want more.		

YOUR METABOLIC FLEXIBILITY SCORE

0—Your metabolism can do full splits!

1–2—Your metabolism can touch its toes but it takes some effort.

3+—Your metabolism needs help getting up from the couch.

As you begin your Reset journey, you will find that these answers will change. As you reset your liver again later this year or next year, remember to redo the quiz after each time because your score will likely move down several points each time.

A BRAND-NEW APPROACH

The Metabolism Reset Diet is a new approach because it addresses the root cause of a slow or inflexible metabolism—an overloaded liver.

The primacy of the liver helps explain why low-fat, low-carb, and ketogenic diets have no special advantage over one another. If you restrict one type of fuel and add more, nothing is gained. For people with poor liver function, sorting out "good" from "bad" food is merely a distraction.

But if this is not a plan of food restriction, what do you eat? How does it work?

During the four weeks, you still eat plenty of good food, but you will do so in ways that help your liver get rid of triglycerides. Triglycerides are temporarily stored dietary fat, fat waiting to be burned as fuel or to get stored long-term as adipose tissue. Think of triglycerides as fats in purgatory.

The Metabolism Reset Diet will help you get rid of high concentrations of triglycerides by eating simple foods in the right ratios at the right times of the day.

The daily schedule is: one smoothie for breakfast, a second smoothie for lunch, one hearty dinner, and snacks as needed. It's that simple. You may be hungry the first few days but by then your liver will already be more capable of giving your body fuel as you need it. Usually, by the first four to six days, you will be less hungry than before starting, which is often a surprise because you are eating less—but the foods you're eating are actually delivering to you the nutrients you need to heal and thrive.

Many people stop me here. It's too hard. I don't have time. I have a full-time job and a family and I can barely keep up with the demands of my life as it is. To this I say: the plan we've devised is probably easier than whatever you're doing now. You will learn how to use liver-friendly foods to make delicious smoothies and meals in no time. Metabolism Reset is perfect when you are busy or traveling, because the Reset menu takes less time and thought than most everyday foods do.

Which foods keep your metabolism working? Thankfully, the list is long and includes vegetables like beets, cabbage, dandelion greens, and shiitake mushrooms; good fats like pumpkin seeds, pistachios, and almonds; carbs with resistant starch like winter squash, boiled potatoes, and navy beans; and lean proteins like salmon, clams, tempeh, and poultry.

Culinary spices will also play an important role. We will make use of turmeric, garlic, basil, and ginger. By converting two of your meals into smoothies, your liver will have a chance to rest and heal.

You will have options that can work with any budget and foods that you can find in any grocery store. If you are cooking for the whole family, they will also love the recipes—my family does. For those who want to undertake a culinary adventure, you will also learn about a few optional exotic ingredients. Everyone can follow the Metabolism Reset Diet, even if you have food intolerances or if you are currently vegan or paleo.

EXERCISE ON THE RESET

The Metabolism Reset Diet exercise plan focuses on light walking, occasional stretching, and three micro workouts weekly, each lasting five minutes or less. If exercise has been a struggle, you are in luck. On the other hand, if you love your hard workouts, expect to do much less than usual during the Reset. But do not fear. You will come back stronger, leaner, and better able to produce energy.

Exercise can keep you from losing too much muscle when you lose fat. The right amounts can boost your mood, lower your cravings, and improve your sleep. However, too much exercise will force your liver to process so much extra fuel and energy, it will never be able to heal. It helps to exercise during the 4 weeks, but you will likely be surprised at how little it takes for the program to work best.

THE END OF FATIGUE

Your energy levels and your weight are related. When your liver does not have enough fuel for short-term energy storage, you feel tired. You don't want to exercise and if you force yourself to, you will hate every minute of it. When your liver gets healthy again, you will have more energy. You will want to do more with your friends, you will look forward to physical activities, and you will wake up more refreshed.

If you haven't felt like yourself lately—maybe even for years—the Metabolism Reset Diet will help you get back on track by reducing dietary fuel intake while giving the liver all of the essential nutrients it needs. In four short weeks, you will be able to store energy temporarily without making it into body fat. Your weight and energy levels will remain steady despite the normal fluctuations in food and activity.

Imagine no longer dieting, restricting, going without. Yes, it is still important to eat good foods, but you'll be able to choose foods that make you feel good, instead of restricting to lose weight.

chapter two

Your Liver Holds the Key

The key to good health is a good metabolism, and the key to a good metabolism is a healthy liver. In this chapter, I take you on a journey of discovery through the secret life of your liver.

LIVER 101: THE BASICS

We marvel at the wonders of the human brain, the ever-beating heart, and the seeming code of destiny, our DNA. But it's the liver that makes the whole show run from backstage. The word *liver* itself comes from the same origin as the word *life*. You cannot live without your liver, in biology or in etymology, and yet we take it for granted every day.

The Greeks called the liver *hepatikos*, which is why we call liver inflammation *hepatitis* and liver cells *hepatocytes*. Today, we think of the brain and the heart as the centers of awareness and emotion, but nearly all ancient cultures saw the liver as the center of both. Traditional medical systems, including the Greek, East Indian, and Chinese, also saw the liver as the main determinant of health. Since the 1800s, naturopathic medicine has placed liver support as step one in managing nearly any chronic illness. Even the newer integrative and functional medical systems understand its importance.

One of many unique things about the liver is its ability to regenerate. Up to 80 percent of your liver can regrow, if damaged. Healthy people can donate over two-thirds of their livers to someone in need—the rest grows back in a matter of months.[1] Consider this fact as a reason for hope. Even if your liver is working poorly now, it can be new and shiny in no time.

WHERE IT IS AND WHAT IT DOES

Your liver sits at the top your abdomen, just beneath your lungs and diaphragm. It is usually larger on the right side, but it reaches all the way to the left. All the blood from your intestinal tract, along with the rest of the blood from your veins, flows through your liver before going back to your heart.[2] Approximately once every minute, your liver filters your entire blood supply.

Can you imagine drinking an eight-ounce glass of water every five seconds nonstop, day and night? That is exactly what your liver constantly does with your blood. Think of your liver as your body's ultimate buffer: it stores, filters, converts, and protects.

STORAGE

Your liver holds on to vitamins, minerals, immune cells, modified amino acids, fuel, and hormones. Think of it as your personal 24-hour grocery store/pharmacy. Some of the micronutrients it stores include B_{12}, iron, copper, vitamin A, vitamin D, and vitamin K. Eating liver is incredibly healthy because it is so high in nutrients: animals' livers store the nutrients just like ours do.[3]

FILTER

The earliest forms of life on earth relied on ocean water for nourishment and chemical stability. If something was not right in the water, life had to move on or adapt if it could. The liver regulates the ecosystem in our bodies, creating a safe little aquarium within our skin. Think of your liver as the filter in the aquarium.

CONVERSION

There are many essential nutrients we can get only from food. Yet there are countless more important nutrients you aren't aware of because your liver quietly builds them for you. These are the nonessential nutrients and conditionally essential nutrients. The only reason we do not call them "essential" is that we know our livers are looking out for us.[4] Examples of these include important amino acids like arginine, glutamine, tyrosine, cysteine, glycine, proline, serine, ornithine, alanine, asparagine, and aspartate.

Amino acids are to your body what individual blocks are to a Lego creation. There are nine amino acids that we have to get from food, but the liver makes the rest. It uses these twenty Legos to make everything solid in your body, as well as countless functional proteins. The liver also regulates your fuel and hormones, and rids the blood of toxicants. In fact, if the liver slacks off even a bit, the poor brain shuts down due to toxicity in the blood, as in the case of hepatic encephalopathy.[5]

Most hormones are made in an inactive state in amounts way above what you need, so that your liver can sort out the details. Imagine that your body is trying to collapse a tunnel in a mountain. It brings lots of dynamite, but your liver lights the sticks after it decides how many sticks to use.

This analogy applies to your thyroid hormones, adrenal stress hormones, reproductive hormones, blood sugar regulating hormones—pretty much everything that is important. In the case of your thyroid, 80 percent or more of its hormones are never used. Your liver turns them into an inactive hormone called reverse T3 and throws them out.[6]

It may sound wasteful, but just like your intake of calories never matches your day's needs, neither do your hormones. In fact, it takes six weeks or more for your thyroid to adjust its output. It is your liver that manages the day-to-day levels by deciding how much to use and how much to waste. If your liver does not manage the thyroid hormones properly, it can slow your metabolism by hundreds of calories per day. Thyroid disease and liver diseases of all types overlap to an alarming degree.[7]

One more example would be your stress hormones. The adrenals mostly make a weak hormone called cortisone. It is mostly up to your liver to make the stronger version, called cortisol, as it sees fit.[8] When this process does not work right, visceral fat grows faster.[9]

Conversion is also essential for getting rid of wastes. Some of these are by-products of our body's daily reactions, like the exhaust from a car. Others come to the liver from the gut bacteria. The liver did not evolve to process drugs or environmental toxicants, but it uses its same tools of conversion to do its best.[10]

LIVER AS PROTECTOR

You may know that a large part of your immune system is governed by intestinal bacteria. However, the intestinal tract is separate from the rest of your body. Guess who is the guard at the gate? Nearly everything entering your body from the intestines must pass through the liver before it gets in.

Your liver is filled with special immune cells called Kuepfer cells. They serve as sentinels and attack anything bad trying to get in. They alert the rest of immunity to the situation on the front lines.[11]

A FUEL'S JOURNEY

Your body burns a little bit of fuel constantly, but it receives a lot of fuel at once, with each meal. If it were not for your liver's ability to store fuel and release it gradually, none of your internal systems could work.

Your liver stores fuel in two forms: glycogen and triglycerides. When it is healthy, it keeps a supply of each fuel, with room to take on more of each. Triglycerides are the ultimate version of stored fuel. The liver can make them out of anything—carbs, fats, ketones, even alcohol. They also store a lot of energy and don't take up much room.

Glycogen is more particular. It can be made only out of carbohydrates and contains much less energy. It has an advantage over triglycerides—the energy stored in glycogen is more readily available. It is easier to burn triglycerides for fuel when you have some glycogen to get the fire started. Think about triglycerides as coals and glycogen as lighter fluid.

Here is where things can go wrong. When the liver is overloaded with too much triglycerides, there is no more room for glycogen. Without glycogen, it is hard to burn triglycerides for fuel, effectively clearing them out. When a load of new fuel comes in from the last meal and the liver is already clogged, all it can do is jam in even more triglycerides or send the fuel away to get stored as body fat.

An overloaded liver also prevents your fat cells from breaking down by making itself resistant to insulin that would otherwise cause the liver to take on more fuel. When the liver is sensitive to insulin, the cells can open up to let in glucose and amino acids. Eventually, fat cells also get filled up and the triglycerides have nowhere to go. Like an airplane that has to circle a crowded airport waiting for an available runway, the triglycerides stay in circulation. Sadly, they are not harmless. In excess, they can damage blood vessels and nerves.

That is what creates a slow metabolism: a liver that is too overloaded to be able to store fuel temporarily.

Eating less does give your liver less fuel to process, which helps. However, it doesn't solve the situation, because eating less can also deprive the liver of the essential nutrients it needs to remove triglycerides. When you do lose fat to supply energy, your liver still has to be ready to take on fuel from the fat cells so that the body can use it gradually.

The other problem is that fat cells are waste dumps. Many environmental pollutants, like solvents, pesticides, and plastic residues, get stuck in them. When your body breaks down fat cells, you send many of these wastes into the liver. This burden of chemicals taxes the same resources your liver would otherwise use to break down triglycerides.

Ultimately, it does not matter if your fuel comes from carbs, dietary fat, ketones, body fat, or alcohol. When there is too much fuel, it becomes triglycerides. When there are too many triglycerides, they clog the liver, increase body fat, and cause disease.[12]

PROTEIN, KETONES, AND ALCOHOL

Protein, ketones, and alcohol are different from fats and carbs in a few ways worth mentioning.

PROTEIN

Protein can be used as fuel, but it does work differently. Protein is the least apt to clog your liver for a number of reasons:

- Protein can act as glycogen and help burn triglycerides.[13]
- Protein has the strongest effect on reducing appetite.[14]
- High-quality protein contains essential amino acids that support the liver's ability to burn triglycerides.[15]
- Protein has the greatest effect on boosting metabolism.[16]

The Metabolism Reset Diet is engineered to provide enough protein for your liver to clear itself out without the need to break down your muscle tissue.

KETONES

Your liver makes ketones when it cannot burn triglycerides. This happens when your blood glucose is low, glycogen is gone, and you cannot break down muscle fast enough. This can happen with a high fat-ketogenic diet because the diet does not supply enough carbs or protein. The ketones made inside your liver are called endogenous ketones.

Some foods have ketones also; these are called exogenous ketones. Medium-chain triglycerides and about 8 to 10 percent of coconut oil can be used as ketones. Wherever they originate, ketones are still fuel, but they are the only form that your liver cannot burn. If your cells are not burning ketones, your liver's only option is to make them into triglycerides, which can clog the liver and form adipose.[17]

Ketones do not cause weight loss. They are just signs of the body's inability to burn triglycerides. On a low-fuel diet, small amounts of ketones are normal. On a ketogenic diet, high amounts of ketones are in the blood and the urine because the body can no longer process ketones—it is just like high blood glucose during insulin resistance.

A large study compared the fat loss from a group on a ketogenic diet against another group on the same amount of fuel from carbs and sugar. When calories were matched, the group eating 25 percent sugar and 50 percent carbs burned more fat than the group on the ketogenic diet.[18] Visit Chapter 10 ("FAQ") for more on ketones.

ALCOHOL

Alcohol from alcoholic beverages itself can serve as fuel after your liver makes it into acetate. However, acetate forms acetaldehyde, which damages liver cells and is a known carcinogen. We call fatty liver "nonalcoholic fatty liver" because the same thing happens to alcoholics. Of all types of fuel, alcohol is most prone to overfill the liver with triglycerides.

OTHER LIVER STRESSORS

We have discussed fuel overload as the main cause of a clogged liver, but a few other factors can contribute. These other factors include an overload of toxicants and a lack of essential dietary nutrients.

TOXICANTS

Your liver is able to process thousands of modern chemicals without a glitch. Some we ingest on purpose, like drugs or food additives. Others creep in without our intent. Yet the liver can easily become overloaded from too much of any one chemical, or too many chemicals at once.

Some toxicants specifically make the liver unable to break down triglycerides. Scientists call the process "toxicant associated steato hepatitis" (TASH). The identified culprits include many chemicals that are common parts of modern life, such as polyvinyl chloride, aflatoxin, trichloroethylene, or tetrachloroethylene. Although these may sound exotic, you are constantly exposed to these chemicals and many others. They come from indoor air, our food, our water, and cosmetics, and get routed straight to our livers.

The heavy metal lead occasionally makes the news as being a contaminant in water. The stories rarely mention that the tap water in up to one-third of homes in America contains unsafe levels of lead and 34 percent still have lead-based paint.[19] Like lead, chloroform is also common in the tap water in many areas. It is also an additive in many sodas, even natural ones—even though you will not see it on the ingredient list.

PCBs (polychlorinated biphenyls) are found in animal fat, farmed salmon, and paints and inks. Whenever a cashier hands you a freshly printed receipt, your liver gets another dose of PCBs that slow your metabolism.[20]

Dioxin is highly concentrated in butter and meat. Shockingly, there is even more dioxin in grass-fed meat and dairy than in commercial meat and dairy.[21] Plastic shopping bags, bottled water, and air in parking lots can expose you to PVC (polyvinyl chloride).[22]

Despite the clear fact that these toxicants can harm our livers in ways that hurt our metabolism, the effects tend not to show up on traditional tests of liver function. The reactions are also more severe by chemicals in combination than from their individual effects, and more pronounced in those with any combination of adiposity, alcohol intake, or prescription medication usage.[23] This means that if you have adiposity, you cannot detox as well and if you can't detox, you get adiposity.

The intestinal tract can also contribute to the load of toxicants on the liver. During constipation, toxic wastes spend too long in the large intestine, and many are absorbed back into the bloodstream and sent straight to the liver. Wastes in the intestinal tract can be bound up by fiber or chlorophyll from green plants, or broken down by good bacteria. When these mitigating factors are not present, it means more work for your liver and more chance of clogging.[24]

THE OUTLOOK FOR DETOXIFYING

As scary as the burden of chemicals can sound, the good news is that the more you detox, the better your body gets at detoxifying. This happens because your liver can process a set amount of chemicals on a daily basis. The fewer new chemicals you give it each day, the more of a chance it has to work on your backlog of toxicants.

The Metabolism Reset Diet includes recipes to help your liver chip away at any stored wastes. It will also teach you how to lower your day-to-day burden of toxicants on your liver.

MISSING NUTRIENTS

Because your liver is involved with so many chemical reactions, nearly all nutrients essential to your body are essential to your liver. However, many people can be lacking in key nutrients their livers need like magnesium,[25] selenium, zinc, vitamin D, vitamin B_{12},[26] folate,[27] vitamin A, lysine, tryptophan,[28] and DHA.[29]

Nutrients supply the raw materials for antioxidants, which can help your liver rid itself of chemicals. Glutathione and superoxide dismutase are made by your liver and are far more powerful than antioxidants from supplements. When your liver cannot make its own antioxidants, it becomes more vulnerable to toxicants and more apt to get clogged.[30]

Along with vitamins and minerals, plant foods provide phytonutrients, which help the liver work better. Some phytonutrients like broccoli, blueberries, or green tea are well documented to help your liver. The Metabolism Reset Diet will lower your chemical burden and give your liver all the nutrients and phytochemicals it needs to give you back your metabolism.

A CLOGGED LIVER

Now that you know how important your liver is, you can see why a clogged liver can cause so many issues in your body. Blood cannot get through easily, it cannot detox, and it drops the ball on the management of the body's hormones, nutrients, and immunity. Along with liver disease, this process is the root of most other chronic diseases.[31]

How would someone feel when his or her liver started getting clogged? Some common symptoms include:

- Feeling tense or stressed
- Moodiness
- Nausea
- Erratic appetite
- Gas and bloating
- Alternating constipation and diarrhea

- Tinnitus
- Bitter taste in the mouth
- Insomnia
- Irritability
- Headaches

These symptoms can be caused by other conditions, yet in the absence of other explanations, the liver is often overlooked.

FROM CLOGGED LIVER TO LIVER DISEASE

When your liver does not work right, it can also develop diseases of its own. Here are some risk factors for liver diseases. If several apply to you, please discuss the concern with your health-care practitioner.

Risk factors—current or previous:

- Mid-body weight gain
- Environmental toxicant exposure
- Ongoing use of prescription medications
- Use of large numbers of supplements

- High blood pressure
- Sleep apnea
- Hepatitis A
- Daily alcohol use
- Thyroid disease
- Gallbladder disease

Blood tests results:

- Morning fasting blood sugar over 90
- Morning fasting insulin level over 10 mlU/L
- Blood level of ALT over 18 U/L females, over 30 males

- Blood level of GGT over 30 U/L in either gender
- Elevated cholesterol
- Elevated triglycerides

Symptoms:

- Fluid retention
- Abdominal distention or bloating
- Jaundice
- Red palms
- Erratic appetite
- Pain or discomfort in the right upper abdomen
- Right shoulder pain
- New allergies/ intolerances
- Dark circles under the eyes
- Breast tenderness (women or men)
- Gynecomastia—enlarged breasts (men)
- Spider angiomas
- Itchy skin
- Easy bruising
- Nosebleeds or prolonged bleeding
- Adult acne
- Dark spots on the skin
- Sensitive to strong odors
- Prone to headaches or migraines
- Eyes red or dry
- Burning sensation in mouth
- Metallic taste in mouth

Liver Disease

If a clogged liver gets bad enough, it goes through four stages of disease progression.

STAGE 1: NAFL

Once the liver gets badly clogged, it can no longer process fuel efficiently and extra triglycerides can make up between 5 and 10 percent of the liver's weight. This is called "steatosis" and nonalcoholic fatty liver disease (NAFL) has started. When steatosis is bad enough, it can cause a faster rate of liver cell death, which shows up on blood tests.

Of the many blood markers of liver function, ALT is the one that matters most for NAFL. ALT means "alanine transaminase." It is a liver enzyme that converts the amino acid alanine to compounds used for energy production. Normally ALT is kept within liver cells, but when they die, ALT spills into the bloodstream. Some ALT in the bloodstream is a normal sign of the liver replacing old cells. However, when ALT is higher, it means cells are dying too quickly.

How high is too high? Surprisingly, one can have an ALT level that is in the "normal" range and still have a problem. Liver specialists agree that the normal range is too broad. Most labs consider ALT levels normal as high as 43 IU/L or even 60 IU/L, yet for adults they should not be higher than 30 IU/L.[32] Other factors like viral hepatitis, medication reactions, or autoimmune hepatitis can raise ALT levels. Once the other factors have been ruled out, NAFL is the most common suspect. The ALT levels often show that NAFL is present but they do not always show how bad it is.

How many people have NAFL? We do not know because the only way to be certain is with a liver biopsy. These are not done for screening purposes with one exception—liver donors. When healthy people offer to donate liver tissue, a biopsy is the only way to be sure their livers are good enough to share. In these situations, 40.2 percent of seemingly healthy potential liver donors have been turned away because they had NAFL. For this reason, many feel that upwards of 40 percent of healthy American adults may have undiagnosed NAFL.[33]

STAGE 2: NASH

When liver cells become too full of fats, eventually they may end up with inflammation within the liver cells.[34] This second stage is called nonalcoholic steatohepatitis (NASH), which simply means the liver cells are inflamed from too much fat. About 10 to 40 percent of those with NAFL eventually progress to NASH.

STAGE 3: FIBROSIS

If inflammation progresses long enough, scar tissue forms and the liver cells suffer irreversible damage. This third state is called hepatic fibrosis. If more than 30 percent of the liver's cells are scarred, the damage is often visible on medical ultrasounds or CT scans.

STAGE 4: CIRRHOSIS

From here, liver function can be so impaired it can be life-threatening. Over time, 25 percent of those with NASH will progress to the fourth stage, called cirrhosis. It is predicted to be one of the leading causes of death in the coming decades.

Don't get too worried just yet—remember, your liver is one of the most resilient organs in your body! Let's shift our discussion to the science behind the liver's ability to repair itself.

THE SUGAR YOU MADE

Because your liver manages your body's fuel supply, further research has shown that it has a large role to play in diabetes. We used to think Type 2 diabetes was an error that made the person's cells ignore the insulin. It turns out that diabetes is primarily a disease of the liver, like adiposity. In fact, some scientists refer to the cause of Type 2 diabetes as "leaky liver."[35] Here is what that means:

Insulin regulates blood sugar in several ways besides just helping it go into the cells. It acts as a brake to stop your liver from converting its glycogen into blood glucose. After a meal with carbs, the carbs provide a source of blood glucose. Carbs also stimulate the release of insulin so that cells can use the glucose. This insulin burst should stop the liver from making glucose.

A clogged liver is so full of extra fuel, it keeps on making glucose because it has no room for glycogen. Furthermore, it doesn't stop making glucose in response to insulin hormone, like a normally functioning liver.[36] In fact, even if a Type 2 diabetic eats a high-carb meal, most of the high blood sugar comes from their liver.[37]

Case Study: Karen

Karen came to see my team for a second opinion on her thyroid care. Like she hoped, my doctors found several ways Karen's thyroid treatment could be improved. They also discovered that she had fatty liver syndrome and was close to being diabetic. Both these issues are exceedingly common. Unfortunately, it is also common that they can go unnoticed or unmentioned by other doctors for years.

The new doctor suggested the Metabolic Reset as the main treatment for both these new findings. Karen's liver function and blood sugar both improved dramatically. Her liver enzymes went from being above normal at 88 U/l to well within optimal range at 13 U/l. Her blood sugar went from borderline diabetes at 6.3 percent down to high-normal at 5.6 percent.

Karen's story was especially memorable because her prior doctor could not believe her lab tests could change so much so quickly and insisted that she repeat them. The repeat labs a month later showed an even greater degree of improvement!

chapter three

Heal Your Liver

You learned in the last chapter that your liver is a superstar, that a clogged liver means a poor metabolism, and that the liver can heal given the right circumstances. In this chapter, I explain what those circumstances are and how they work together in a four-week program. Here is the science behind the Metabolism Reset.

There are two essential steps to opening up a clogged liver:

Step 1: The Liver Repair Diet
- High conjugation
- Low fuel

Step 2: Body Reset
- Sleep debt payoff
- Micro workouts

STEP 1: THE LIVER REPAIR DIET

HIGH CONJUGATION

A *conjugation* is more than a part of speech we learn in English class. *Conjugation* means "to join up" or "to bond together." Your liver needs conjugating nutrients in order to get rid of fat and toxicants.

The liver cleans itself in a two-phase process: activation and conjugation. Imagine a mining operation. The goal is to get the coal out of the ground. First, you have to break the coal off the wall, and then you have to put the coal in a cart to haul it out.

In the activation phase, wastes are "activated," or chemically altered, so they are ready to stick to something. This phase is like your body's chipping coal from the wall. During conjugation, that waste is packaged up in certain nutrients so that it can be sent out of the body without making trouble along the way. This is like the coal going into the cart.[1] The conjugation phase is performed by amino acids, stimulated by phytonutrients, and aided by dietary fibers. The more your liver needs to detox, the faster this process goes. The problem is that lots of things speed up activation more than conjugation: caffeine, alcohol, environmental chemicals, you name it. Often it goes too fast for conjugation to keep up.

This is why fasting is not always effective for detoxifying. Fasting does cause wastes to move out of where they are stored, but because your liver doesn't have enough material for conjugation, the wastes often end up leaving the tissues and moving right back into the bloodstream. From there, they hit your liver again and might even relocate to the brain.[2]

Diets high in phytonutrients assist the liver's ability to eliminate wastes and process fuel more efficiently. The best way to help an overactive pathway during the activation phase appears to be by eating a combination of cruciferous vegetables such as broccoli, cauliflower, and cabbage in conjunction with apiaceous vegetables like carrots, parsley, and parsnips. Women's livers respond to these foods even better than men's livers do.[3]

There are also great foods that speed up the conjugation phase to help it keep up. These boost the liver's internal defenses like NrF2 and glutathione, and include fish, turmeric, tomatoes, papaya, garlic, onions, radishes, grapes, and soy products.[4, 5, 6, 7]

FIBERS, OR NOT FIBER?

We think of fiber as one thing when really it is a category of things. For fibers, variety is important, just like it is for every other part of the diet. Your intestinal bacteria are fed by different types of fibers. The total quantity of fiber matters, but emerging studies suggest that fiber diversity is just as essential.

The Metabolism Reset provides a variety of fibers by including all categories of fiber-rich plant foods: legumes, intact whole grains, nuts, seeds, vegetables, and fruits.

Remember that conjugation depends on amino acids from protein. You can get the amino acids that your liver cannot make itself from any food rich in protein, but some of the conjugating superstars include poultry, pumpkin seeds, mollusks, lentils, mung beans, sunflower seeds, and white beans.[8]

The Metabolism Reset provides an abundance of food-derived conjugating factors and aids to help your liver clear out the gunk that is clogging it.[9]

LOW FUEL

Since all fuel has to be processed by your liver, the Reset uses a low-fuel formula to help create space for triglycerides. Once you make room for them, you can start breaking down adipose tissue again.

By fuel, I mean any combination of carbs, fats, or ketones. In this situation, I prefer the term "fuel" rather than "calories." That's because not all calories are the same. Those from protein and resistant starch are processed differently from those from fats and carbs. I also think we have gotten too hung up in a battle between carbs, fats, and ketones. As far as an overloaded liver is concerned, they're all treated equally as fuel.

IS IT FUEL OR IS IT JUST CALORIES?

The calorie is likely the most divisive source of energy we consume. The truth is that, when test subjects are in controlled settings, a surplus of calories causes weight gain while a deficit of calories causes weight loss, regardless of where the calories come from.

Calories are real, but the calorie model alone does not perfectly predict every individual's weight. You can gain fat on fresh greens, wild-caught salmon, and organic blueberries—if you eat enough of them. Bears do it every winter.

For further proof on the power of calories, you can drop weight, reverse diabetes, and lower blood pressure on a diet of Oreos, Doritos, and Twinkies—as long as you watch your calorie count.[10] Mind you, who knows what such a diet would do if it were carried out long term? Would the number of random chemicals you would ingest create more risk than the benefits of weight loss?

GIVING CALORIES NUANCE

The calorie model is hard to apply universally because of variations in a given person's metabolism, and the roles of protein and resistant starch.

Variations in metabolism come in two forms: deviations from expected metabolic rate, and range of metabolic flexibility. The basal metabolic rate (BMR) is how many calories you burn each day just keeping your body warm and carrying out basic maintenance. For anyone exercising under eight hours per day, this is by far the biggest source of calories burned. It is governed almost exclusively by how much lean body mass you have, your gender, and your age—in that order.

You can estimate your BMR or you can measure it. I have seen first-hand that people of the same size, gender, and age can have a threefold range in BMR when accurately measured. Those with the lowest BMR are ones who say they barely eat and gain weight, while those with the highest BMR are those who eat more and stay thin.

Metabolism can also vary in terms of metabolic flexibility. Your body has the ability to keep your weight steady and keep your body functioning, despite changes in your fuel intake from food and your fuel output from physical activity, also known as net calories. Net calories are the calories you consume after subtracting the extra calories burned from physical work or exercise. If you eat 1800 calories and burn 200 calories from exercise, your net calories for the day are 1600 calories (1800 − 200 = 1600).

All of us have a range of net calories where eventually, if we consume too much fuel, we will gain weight. If we burn off too much fuel, we will lose weight and feel the need to rest. Say that Cindy can stay trim and feel fine as long as she eats anywhere between 1300 and 2000 net calories per day. You can say that she has a flexible metabolism. However, say that Anna loses weight only if she goes below a net amount of 1300 calories; but when she does, she feels miserable. She cannot deal with people and she has unrelenting food cravings. But if she raises her food up to just 1500 net calories, her weight starts going up. Anna does not have a flexible metabolism.

The sad fact is that there are scores of people just like Anna. These are people who will not be able to lose a pound until they starve themselves to a point at which they feel rotten. But by unclogging your liver, you can reset your metabolism and experience that same flexibility that Cindy does.

The low-fuel diet is structured to give you optimal protein so that you conjugate well, keep your muscles intact, and feel energized along the way. Optimal protein is the difference between removing adipose tissue for good and going on a yo-yo diet.[11] The number 3 is the magic number on a low-fuel diet. Each day you will have 3 protein servings and 3 fuel servings from 2 shakes, 1 meal, and unlimited veggie snacks. The fuel will come from good carbs and healthy fats.

CARBS

If your goal is metabolic flexibility, carbs are a tool that can help when used carefully. A diet that is too low in good carbs blocks your liver from burning triglycerides. Carbs also help your liver make glutathione,[12] activate thyroid hormones,[13] lower cortisol,[14] and feed your good bacteria.[15]

This combination makes them a bad fit for those trying to reset their metabolism. At the other end of the spectrum, a diet high in processed carbs may be harder for glycemic regulation in those in the diabetes continuum. For that reason, it's just not safe.

There are plenty of benefits to a moderate intake of carbs, especially fibers and resistant starch, along with the production of glycogen. A higher intake of fibers is good for conjugation because it keeps the wastes in your colon from going back to your liver again and again.[16] Good carbs can also be sources of phytonutrients that help your liver.

Here are some of the best examples:

- Adzuki beans
- Beets
- Black beans
- Blueberries
- Buckwheat
- Dark cherries
- Lentils
- Pomegranate seeds
- Purple potatoes
- Quinoa
- Squash
- Sweet potatoes (yams)
- Turnips
- Wild rice

RESISTANT STARCH

Resistant starch (RS) has a whole host of benefits, such as:

- Improved liver function
- Better regulation of blood sugar
- Repair of metabolic syndrome
- Reduction of visceral fat
- Reduced adiposity
- Improved muscle mass
- Healthier gut flora[17,18]

Where can we get resistant starch in our diets? The food category with the highest amount of it by far is legumes. Often you hear "beans" and "legumes" as if they were interchangeable terms. In truth, legumes are a larger category that includes beans, chickpeas (garbanzo beans), carob, lentils, mesquite, and peas.

In a study that tracked over 10,000 participants for nine years, 1 ounce of legumes with RS each day lowered mortality more than any other food group. And 1 ounce of beans lowered the death risk by more than 8.5 ounces of vegetables.[19]

Another study tested whether legumes could help menopausal women shrink their waists and improve their liver function. They tracked two groups of women on the same diet, with the same number of calories. One group's diet included some hidden legumes. No one knew which diet they were on. Within just a few weeks, it became apparent that those getting the hidden legumes got thinner and had healthier livers. They also had lasting improvement in cholesterol and blood pressure.[20]

People often do not eat enough legumes, owing to fears of phytonutrients like lectins and phytates. However, the evidence is clear: those who eat legumes are healthier than those who do not.

Since RS is a type of carbohydrate, it is also found in a few other foods with good carbs. In addition to legumes, other examples of resistant starches include:

- Bananas/plantains
- Beans
- Grains
- Potatoes
- Supplement sources

FATS

In the four-week program, healthy fats are included to provide essential fatty acids and accessory nutrients. The type of fats we choose can also reduce inflammation and insulin sensitivity. Like carbs, fats can supply helpful nutrients, or they can lead to fuel overload.

First, let us define "essential fatty acid." There are only two: linoleic acid, also called omega-6, and linolenic acid, also called omega-3. These are also *polyunsaturated* fatty acids, which come from cold-water fish, nuts, and seeds. *Monounsaturated* fats are those in Mediterranean foods, like olive oil, almonds, and avocados. These fats are not essential, but they are a good neutral source of fuel.

Finally, there are *saturated* fats. These are not essential and can be completely harmless in low amounts: roughly 7 to 10 percent of your total calories. For years, we mistakenly thought that even small amounts of them, like 3 to 5 percent, could cause heart disease. But when science showed this was not the case, many people went too far and started treating saturated fats like superfoods. They are not villains, but they are also not superfoods.

When our intake of saturated fat goes well above 15 or 20 percent, it makes our cell membranes less fluid and clumpy. Imagine butter or lard sitting on your counter next to olive oil. The fats that are most saturated flow less easily, and the same is true in your cells. High intakes of saturated fats are linked with diabetes,[21] breast cancer,[22] and premature brain aging.[23]

We also have *trans fatty* acid, which is totally harmful, with no benefits. It is even outlawed in many countries. Trans fatty acid is formed by heating polyunsaturated fatty acids or monounsaturated fatty acids to high levels. It is also naturally occurring in fat from dairy and beef, which is why the Metabolism Reset relies on cold-water fish, nuts, seeds, and vegetables for its fats.

PROTEIN

When it comes to healing your metabolism, protein is different from fats and carbs. You can do fine for a while on less fuel from fats and carbs, but your body still needs just as much protein.

Protein is the sole source of the essential amino acids your liver needs to conjugate wastes and triglycerides. Diets without abundant essential amino acids, from high-quality protein foods, do not allow for optimal liver conjugation.[24]

Like fats and carbs, protein has been the topic of much misinformation. I often see or hear statements like: "We don't need that much protein," or "You cannot get a protein deficiency," or "Americans die from eating too much protein." It is true that minimal protein needs are easy to meet. It is also true that highly processed animal foods like sausage and bacon create substantial risks to those who overconsume them.

Let's distinguish between minimal protein needs and optimal protein needs while on a low-fuel diet. The recommended daily intake of protein is pretty low. A 140-pound woman can eat as little as 50 grams (roughly 2 servings) per day and prevent a deficiency.[25] Yet when we lower food intake for any reason, protein intake normally goes down dramatically. Your body makes up for the difference by eating up your muscles as a source of protein.

For example, a 140-pound woman has her best chance at reducing adipose tissue and healing her metabolism by including at least 90 grams of protein in her diet.[26] This equals about three generous servings of protein. The four-week program provides this amount in the two shakes and one evening meal.

What's the right amount of protein? Just like all parts of the diet, balance is best. Studies have shown that it is safe to consume over three times the amount of protein as recommended by the Metabolism Reset.[27] The top examples of high-quality protein include:

- Fish
- Lean grass-fed beef
- Mollusks
- Pea protein powder

- Poultry
- Shellfish
- Tempeh

Pea protein has several distinct properties, making it an especially good fit for the Metabolism Reset. As a vegetable protein, it is alkalizing, which means it does not create the acidic burden that animal protein creates. This concern is especially relevant on a low-fuel diet. And unlike hemp or other vegetable proteins, pea protein is able to form a molecular gel when mixed with water, which can improve absorption.[28] Several scientific studies have proved that pea protein is better than other foods at reducing appetite and regulating blood sugar.[29]

Pea protein is also more effective than dairy protein at limiting the amount of triglyceride-forming cholesterol and saturated fat absorbed from the intestinal tract into the liver.[30] Finally, pea protein is a better choice than dairy proteins like whey and casein, because the latter can raise growth hormones, which can prevent the breakdown of stored fat in the liver cells.[31]

UNLIMITED FOODS

What are unlimited foods? Yep, it is as good as it sounds. You can have as much of these foods as you want, whenever you want them. They are unlimited because they provide lots of valuable phytonutrients and an insignificant amount of fuel.

Even if you do not end up snacking on them, it is best to have at least three servings per day between your shakes and meal. Go ahead and chow down.

Here are just a few examples of great unlimited food options:

- Baby carrots
- Bell peppers
- Broccoli
- Celery
- Greens, all kinds
- Tomatoes
- Zucchini

CALORIES FROM PROTEIN AND RESISTANT STARCH

Calories from protein raise metabolism directly, stimulate muscle growth (which also raises metabolism), and are more filling than calories from carbs, fats, or ketones. Another key element of protein is satiety. Optimal-protein diets, from both animal and plant-derived proteins, are effective for lowering appetite in weight-loss programs.[32]

Even though your body shows changes in leptin and ghrelin that would normally raise appetite, protein can keep hunger at bay as long as you are getting optimal amounts. This means that you can get away with eating less and feeling much fuller, without any real negative drawbacks.[33]

In fact, when it comes to your basal metabolic rate, protein raises your metabolism more than any other type of food. Also known as the "thermic effects of food," an optimal-protein diet can raise metabolism by 15 percent.[34] This elevation continues as long as you consume more protein; your body doesn't adjust back to a lower metabolic state as long as you eat enough protein.

At first, low-carb diets seemed to work better at achieving a loss of adipose tissue and lowering appetite. However, researchers have pointed out that most low-carb diets are also high-protein diets. More recent studies have been done to find out if it was a low-carb diet that helped the weight loss, or if it was the high-protein aspects. When researchers control the protein levels, the amount of carbs or fat no longer seems to matter—low-fat high-protein diets work just as well as low-carb high-protein diets.[35] The other case in which calories do not apply equally is that of resistant starch. Starch is a type of carbohydrate made up of large clusters of smaller carbohydrate molecules.

Resistant starch yields only about half the expected calories because it resists digestion. And its benefits extend well beyond the bonus calories. It also stabilizes the blood sugar, and the calories that aren't used are the most powerful fuel known for feeding our good bacteria.

Because of the blood sugar effects, RS helps burn adiposity, lowers diabetes risk, and helps steady the energy levels. Because of its effects on good bacteria, it improves immunity, lowers cancer risks, and improves digestive health.

MICRONUTRIENTS

Low-fuel diets can cause a micronutrient deficiency, however. What's the solution to this problem? The Metabolism Reset ensures adequate levels of micronutrients, by having the focus on eating unprocessed foods from as many categories as possible, avoiding highly processed foods, and judiciously using micronutrient supplementation. Micronutrients are essential for the liver to be able to process trapped fuel and toxins. The modern diet is often too high in fuel and too low in the micronutrients it needs to run all of its detoxification processes.

HOW LONG SHOULD THE LOW-FUEL RESET LAST?

Remember, this is a Reset. After four weeks on the Metabolism Reset, you will still need to watch your total fuel intake and focus on unprocessed foods, but you will be able to maintain your health and weight without needing to be as restrictive. If you complete the four weeks and wish to lose more weight or achieve further changes, you can repeat the Reset up to once every three months or up to four times per year without slowing your metabolism.

FOOD TIMING

The four-week Reset plan encourages regular food timing because the liver works best when the body's daily rhythms are predictable. If you have ever cared for a baby, you may have learned that things go well until the moment the routine gets broken. Think of your liver like a baby. By timing your shakes and meals at regular intervals each day, your energy levels, appetite, and mood will be more manageable, even though your fuel intake is lower.[36]

Between meals, you can eat as needed, and you will have many good options from the unlimited foods list. After the first few days, most people find that they are less hungry and are more content with the shakes and meals.

SHAKES AND MEAL REPLACEMENTS

The Metabolic Reset structures the day around two shakes, one meal, and unlimited snacks. Meal replacement has been shown by numerous studies to be more effective than food restriction.[37] It has been proven to provide many benefits, including:

- Faster initial weight loss
- Greater success on long-term follow-up
- Higher rates of compliance
- Reduced fatty liver
- Reduced waist circumference
- Lowered body fat
- Reduced inflammation[38,39,40]

A study done in 2013 compared the efficacy of meal replacement with either one or two meal shakes per day, using a group of 36 overweight patients with poorly controlled diabetes. Those given two shakes per day lost eight times as much weight as those on a single shake per day. Participants also found the two-shake program just as easy to adhere to as the single shake program.

Two shakes also won out over three shakes per day. When compared to a more restrictive program that allowed three shakes and no solid food, the group using two shakes per day got the same benefits and had an easier time sticking with the program.[41]

Why does meal replacement seem to help? For one, you have fewer decisions to make. There is a concept called *decision fatigue*. It means that the more things you have to think about, the harder it is to make decisions. With the Metabolic Reset, you can make two meals at once in a matter of minutes. It cuts down on making those stressful and frustrating food choices, and it simplifies the process so that it's easier to follow.

It's also the easiest way to get high protein and low fuel. Protein is found in many foods, from animals and plants. However, cutting down on carbs and fats can be hard when most natural sources of protein have a good amount of either fuel. Shakes can be made with protein powder that has no, or minimal, fuel. This way, you get the right amount of protein without ingesting too much carbs or fats.

For example, foods that have protein + fat include:

- Nuts
- Seeds
- Cheese
- Meat
- Dark-meat poultry
- Soy foods

Food that have protein + carbs include:

- Legumes
- High-protein grains (quinoa, winter wheat, amaranth)

THE CASE FOR SHAKES

The evidence on protein shakes is, frankly, staggering. In a controlled study of 100 obese adults, higher-protein meal replacement led to more fat loss and less loss of muscle mass than standard meal replacements, even at the same calorie intake.[42]

Muscle loss is especially dangerous in older adults who are intentionally losing weight. In a double-blind study, with 80 older adults on a low-calorie diet, protein supplementation showed an increase of roughly 1 pound of muscle mass, whereas the group with only dietary protein showed a loss of up to 4 pounds of muscle mass.[43] This is the critical difference in an aging population that can't really afford to lose any muscle tissue.

There have also been studies comparing shakes with food. Tracked for 40 weeks, 90 obese adults were randomized to have either meals or two shakes and one meal. The shakes group lost more weight (12.3 percent body weight vs. 6.9 percent). Additionally, the food group did not have more satiety, while the shake group saw a significant reduction in inflammation and oxidative stress. The best part of this study was that compliance rates were also higher in the shake group than for meal-based weight-loss programs. The fact of the matter is that people didn't get bored with the shakes plan, even when they were using only two flavors of shakes. People preferred using meal replacements, even when they were doing it for 16 straight weeks.

The revolution in meal replacements and shakes has shown that a low-fuel diet can work, helping to unclog the liver in a meaningful way.

STEP 2: BODY RESET

In order for the Metabolism Reset to be as effective as possible, you have two important lifestyle changes to make: paying off your sleep debt, and exercising in "micro workouts."

SLEEP DEBT PAYOFF

Yes, your sleep is important to metabolism, but it is your *total* sleep debt that counts, not just how much sleep you got last night. *Sleep debt* is defined as the total amount of sleep you have missed over time.

Sleep matters because melatonin, the sleep hormone, also helps the liver rebuild its glycogen supplies. More glycogen equals a better metabolism. It turns out that your body is most able to rebuild glycogen and burn stored fat during prolonged deep sleep.[44] Melatonin has also been shown to reverse the exact genetic damage that leads to the spiral of fat buildup.[45]

High-quality sleep is also essential because it prevents the body from releasing high amounts of the fat-loss-blocking cortisol, which can lead to:

- Low mood
- Overwhelming food cravings
- Slower metabolism

Sleep will even help your genes work with you rather than against you. Have you ever thought that your genes were sabotaging your jeans? Even if you have genes that make you prone to gain weight and unable to lose it, the more sleep you get, the less these genes matter.[46]

When you're well-rested, you also make better food decisions. Your brain's insular cortex regulates pleasure-seeking behavior. We all experience signals from our brain, encouraging us to seek out pleasurable experiences, like high-fuel junk food. But does it have to be ice cream? Would a nap work as well? The less sleep debt you have, the more you can choose how you act on these signals for comfort.

How Large Is Your Sleep Debt?

This is a quick quiz so you can learn whether your sleep debt is no big deal, or if it is leading you toward imminent foreclosure. Score one point for each box you check off.

☐ Do you have afternoon food cravings?
☐ Do you need an alarm to wake up?
☐ Do you need caffeine to get going in the morning?
☐ Do you often fall asleep after lunch?
☐ Do you fall asleep when reading?
☐ Do you get irritable interacting with your spouse or family?
☐ Do you find it hard to concentrate?
☐ Do you sleep in on weekends?
☐ Do you fall asleep at random times?

Find out how you scored:

0   Chances are you have no sleep deficit.
1–3   You have a mild sleep deficit. Consider trying to get $8\frac{1}{2}$ hours of sleep during your Reset.
4+   You have a major sleep deficit, and should consider a "sleeping vacation" during the beginning of the Reset process.

What kind of sleep targets should you be shooting for during the Reset process? Figure $7\frac{1}{2}$ hours as the absolute minimum for most people. Some find, with this simple change, that they have less hunger and better energy levels when they get more—$8\frac{1}{2}$ to 9 solid hours of sleep.

THE PERFECT SLEEP VACATION

Sometimes we just need to get away and get some rest. If you are operating with a major sleep deficit, or even a minor one, you might want to consider a sleep vacation to help get that debt paid off. When do you do it? If you have a major sleep deficit, you should consider it at any point in time—it is especially great for the first few days of a Reset.

Book a hotel room for a weekend. Request no television, or just ask them to remove the remote control. Also, request that no snack options are present in the room. Put up the "Do Not Disturb" sign, and turn your phone on airplane mode. And bring supplies for shakes, with protein powder, and an all-in-one meal replacement:

- Multivitamins
- Greens
- Seeds
- Berries
- Stevia

Also, make sure you have lots of water. Hydration is always important, especially when you're on a sleep vacation. And be sure to pre-schedule approved meals from room service. Consider the room-service menu options when choosing a hotel in your area for your vacation, as they should have fish, poultry, steamed vegetables, brown rice, baked potato, or black beans.

If the idea of going off the grid scares you, consider appointing a "sleep guardian." This is kind of like a buddy system, where you have someone who can monitor your phone calls or your email account. Give the person a way to get ahold of you, only if it is absolutely essential.

A sleep vacation might just be your golden ticket to feeling better, and resetting your rhythm so that your liver can do a better job of doing its job.

MICRO WORKOUTS

The final aspect of the Metabolic Reset is the exercise portion called the micro workouts. Why is it that so many people can't seem to lose weight when they exercise hard? Exercise is a beautiful thing when you have a good metabolism. When you do not, though, it is a huge stress on your body. Studies have shown that the reason many people cannot lose weight is that they are exercising too much.[47] Your liver has to process all the fuel you burn when you exercise hard. If it is already having a hard time providing energy, the extra burden just makes things worse.

Some exercise is essential for glycogen production and muscle health. This allows you to unclog your liver by creating more helpful glycogen that can keep things humming. Micro workouts help in this sense because they:

- Help you retain your muscles
- Don't require your liver to process more fuel
- Make your mitochondria stronger

Quick workouts can work better for your metabolism than longer workouts while you are on a low-fuel diet. If it's done right, the workouts also do not raise hunger.[48] Micro workouts are part of the Reset that will heal your metabolism so you can enjoy more food and enjoy more exercise.

THE METABOLIC RESET

The Metabolic Reset is a brief process—all it takes is four weeks. It heals your metabolism so that you can quit the hassles and stress of dieting. It helps take care of your liver, which is your key to metabolic flexibility, by creating more room for glycogen and helping to detox one of the most important parts of your body.

As for the food on this diet? You remain low on fuel while still getting enough protein to keep you going strong. At the same time, you have the opportunity to reset your circadian cycle by paying off your sleep debt. Sleep resets your gene expression, so that the genes of weight gain won't be able to hold you back any longer. The micro workouts are just right enough to energize your muscles and keep your metabolism primed, without stressing your system.

Now that you understand the science of the Metabolic Reset, let's move into the next section and learn how to prepare for the program.

chapter four

Prepare for a New Metabolism

Imagine that in another month from now you feel lighter, more energetic, and are able to stop dieting. These changes have happened to thousands of people before you, and with a little planning, you too will have an effective Reset.

SETTING EXPECTATIONS

A healthy liver and metabolism are the goal, but many also notice the side benefit of losing pounds and inches. Of course, results can vary, but our clinical trial showed that women see an average of $2^1/_2$ inches of waist loss, or 9 pounds of fat loss per Reset.

The more adipose tissue someone has to lose, the more dramatic the Reset can be. Some have lost over 5 inches in the four weeks. The converse is also usually true: those who are closer to their target fat level see fewer total inches lost. There is also a gender difference: women lose more inches, whereas men lose more pounds.

Expect the first one to three days to be a period of adjustment. The more clogged your liver is, the more dramatic this adjustment may be. For most, it is some extra hunger, but some have noticed fatigue, food cravings, headaches, irritability, bloating, and even skin rashes. By day 3, these symptoms should be decreasing. By day 6, you will likely have less hunger, steadier energy, and even more mental clarity than before you started.

When you get into the second week, you can expect to be in a good rhythm with the program. You may even notice that you have more free time than usual, since your meals do not take much thought or preparation and because your workouts are so short. The rest of the remaining time often flies by. You may even be tempted to keep on going after the four weeks are over. Please visit Chapter 10 ("FAQ") for ideas if you find yourself in this situation.

Now that you know what to expect, here are the steps to get you ready.

STEP 1—DETERMINE WHY YOU ARE DOING THIS

Why do you want to improve your health? In other words, why did you pick up this book and not a novel? It may seem that the answers are self-evident. Don't we all want to be thin and healthy? Nonetheless, know that the better you answer this question, the better your Reset will go. It can seem that your motivations are clear—until you put them into words. It may indeed determine how well this program works for you, so here are a few suggestions and prompts to help you answer this question.

RESET JOURNAL

If you already have a personal journal, please use it. If not, get a nice notebook and your favorite pen. You can use it to track your progress, but first take about ten minutes to describe your motivations for starting the program. Here are a few cues to jog your creativity:

PROMPT #1: SELFISH REASONS

Often these seem to be the first reasons that come to mind—and that is okay. Do you want to look better in a swimsuit? Feel more confident in social situations? Have healthier skin? Feel more light and nimble? Have you ever had fantasies about what life would be like if you were thinner? Now is not the time to judge yourself for it; instead, use it for momentum. Feel free to indulge this fantasy and let it play out in your journal.

PROMPT #2: HEALTH BENEFITS

Maybe you would like to have lower cholesterol levels or sleep better. Perhaps you have been tired of taking medications. Maybe you saw how diabetes wrecked the course of a relative's life and you do not want to go that way. What could an effective Metabolism Reset mean to your health?

PROMPT #3: FOR OTHERS

Now that your creative process is engaged, here is the most powerful motivator of all. Your health does not just serve you, it also makes you better for your loved ones. Imagine that you could connect better with your romantic partner or have an easier time finding one. What would that be worth? What if you could play tag with your kids or grandkids? If you had lots of energy left over, how could you help the social causes that matter to you?

Throughout the Reset and after, try to get into the habit of revisiting these reasons to keep yourself connected to what really matters.

STEP 2—LOWER YOUR CHEMICAL BURDEN

The better your liver can function, the better your metabolism will work. One of the reasons many people have lost their metabolic flexibility is due to the chemicals their livers need to process each day. Here are a few steps to give your liver less junk to deal with.

Imagine this chemical burden as a sink that overflows and damages your floor. To prevent this from happening, you make sure the drain is open and the faucet is shut off. In our analogy, the drain represents the body's ability to eliminate waste, and the faucet is the number of chemicals entering it. Unfortunately, it is impossible to reduce your daily chemical exposure down to zero. You cannot shut the faucet off completely, but you can take some simple steps to slow it down to a tiny drip.

Start with your indoor air. As important as it is to secure clean food, many people are surprised to learn that the largest single source of chemical exposure by far is not food but, rather, the air in our homes. The chapters on food will give you ways to lower your intake of chemicals from the diet. But here are some simple action steps you can take right away to reduce your daily chemical burden by 90 percent or more.

From what follows, start with the first pass, then do the quick clean, and finally the deep clean. Make any changes that seem easy, and set a reminder to look at these lists once per month, until you have completed all of the steps. That is, don't get overwhelmed, and don't do nothing—your metabolism is too important for that! Begin with the first pass.

FIRST PASS

- Declare your home a no-shoe zone. Put a rack at the front door, with slippers of various sizes and a sign asking guests to kindly remove their shoes before entering.
- Do not let anyone smoke in or near your home.
- Replace any indoor air fresheners with an essential-oil diffuser. Use blends of pure essential oils or consider individual oils such as cinnamon, wild orange, clove, or sandalwood.
- Shop for unscented detergents and fabric softeners.
- If weather and circumstances allow, start keeping your doors and windows open to outside air as much as possible. Even areas with known air pollution have cleaner air outside than inside many homes.
- Use only purified water for drinking. Reverse-osmosis units are most practical for home usage.

QUICK CLEAN

- Replace your air filters with pleated filters. Look for a minimum efficiency reporting value (MERV) of at least 7. Set a reminder on your calendar to replace your air filters every eight weeks.
- Choose an outdoor space to park clothes from the dry cleaners. Get in the habit of letting them off-gas outside your home for at least three days before putting them in your closet.
- Use a HEPA air filter in your bedroom while you are sleeping. Bear in mind how much cubic footage the unit will treat compared to the size of your bedroom. Sometimes it takes multiple units to treat larger bedrooms. To find the cubic footage of your bedroom, multiply its length by its width by its height. Plan to replace filters on the manufacturer's schedule. HEPA filters also provide white noise, which may improve sleep.
- In your kitchen, replace plastic food containers with glass, steel, and silicone. Use parchment or aluminum foil instead of plastic wrap. Replace nonstick or aluminum cookware with cast iron, stainless steel, or ceramic titanium. As far as I'm concerned, nothing beats well-seasoned cast iron for cooking. It lasts forever, holds heat well, distributes it evenly, and is inexpensive.

DEEP CLEAN

- Replace all kitchen and laundry cleaning chemicals with fragrance-free versions.
- Install an inline water filter on your showerhead to remove chlorine.
- To purify your bathwater and get rid of the chlorine, place a 1-quart jar containing 3 cups bentonite clay and $1/2$ cup powdered vitamin C next to your bathtub with a tablespoon-size

measuring spoon. Shake well. Add 2 tablespoons of the mixture to bathwater and let sit for 10 minutes before bathing.

- Read the labels on all your cosmetics, skin-care items, and hair-care products. Make note of those that contain parabens, PEG, and triclosan, and change to a safer brand immediately or with your next refill.

- Inspect your bathroom and kitchen for any signs of water damage. If you see any, have an environmental engineer evaluate your home for mold.

- Schedule air-duct cleaning at least annually and carpet cleaning at least twice annually.

Case Study: Brad

Brad was a 37-year-old man who came to see me to screen him for mercury toxicity. Brad had seen a news story about a celebrity whose career nearly ended after overdosing on mercury from tuna. Apparently, the celebrity was eating tuna at sushi restaurants several times per week for years, and the mercury buildup led to odd symptoms like tics and tremors that she could not control.

Brad heard the story and flipped because he was having similar symptoms, and he had eaten tuna almost every day for over a decade. If the celebrity had a problem, Brad figured that he must be even worse. Brad's family doctor had tested him for mercury already, but told him he was fine. Brad was so sure he was toxic from mercury, he sought me out as a second opinion.

I explained to Brad how the other doctor's tests were good at detecting mercury from the last few days but they could miss a long buildup over years. We did more sensitivity tests and found out that he did have dangerously high levels of mercury. Over the course of the next few months, I was able to bring Brad's mercury back down to safe levels. On one of his follow-up visits, he asked me if the mercury could have made him fat.

He asked because, in the last few weeks, he had dropped over 12 pounds with no changes in diet or exercise. I explained to him how anything that stresses your liver can slow your metabolism, and that the detox could have helped him shed more than the mercury.

STEP 3—GET YOUR KITCHEN READY

If you want it easy, you got it. The Reset program can be as simple as mixing a pre-made shake in a shaker bottle, munching on baby carrots for snacks, and heating a few things from the supermarket for your meals. In Chapter 5 on food, you will learn how you can spend as little as 15 minutes per day on the whole food process and not need any new equipment.

Plan ahead to be hungry for the first few days, and have some good unlimited snacks ready. The hunger battles are won by planning, not by willpower. Look at the unlimited food recipes and choose a few to have ready on standby. Also, be sure to remove any snack foods that you would not plan to eat during the Reset. It is tempting to think that you will stay out of them. You might even feel like you would be depriving your spouse or kids if the junk were gone. But you wouldn't be. Donate the snacks to a food bank or send them with your spouse to take to work.

Here is a list of some of the highest priority "foods" to banish from your kitchen:

- All dry carbs, such as crackers, chips, popcorn, cookies
- Sweetened cereals
- Salted nuts
- Sweets
- Candy
- Cakes
- Juices and sodas

GATHER YOUR TOOLS

If you love to play and experiment in the kitchen, here are some of my favorite kitchen toys to help engage your inner chef.

HIGH-POWERED BLENDER

You will have the option of adding various greens, seeds, and other additions to your shakes. Nearly any blender can do the job, but the more powerful it is, the smoother the result will be. High-powered blenders have features like pre-programmed cycles based on your ingredients and have covers to muffle the noise. Many of the current generation miniature blenders, like the NutriBullet, even have enough power to do a good job with vegetables.

Note: We had a trusty Vitamix in our kitchen for over 20 years. I was conflicted about spending several hundred dollars on a blender at the time, but we sure got the miles out of it. Recently it seemed to have given up the ghost and we replaced it with a new Blendtec. We all love the difference that the sound enclosure makes. A few days after the new Blendtec arrived, I was tinkering with the old Vitamix and got it working as good as new. The point is this: do not be scared of investing in a good blender, as it will do a much better job on your smoothies and will last forever.

RICE COOKER

Intact whole grains are great sources of RS, fiber, good carbs, B vitamins, and minerals. You can easily steam them on the stovetop with a saucepan, but rice cookers make this job effortless and foolproof. Just add one part grain and two parts water, close the unit, and press "cook." You can walk away and your grains will cook exactly as long as they should, as well as be kept warm until you are ready to eat them. How do they work? Elven magic.

Note: Look for a rice cooker that has a steel cooking container, as opposed to aluminum or nonstick. They also work well for steel-cut oats; just be sure to leave the lid ajar so the liquid does not boil over.

PRESSURE COOKER

If you want to cook food quickly with the most flavor and nutrition possible, pressure cookers are the way to go. They excel at dried beans and tough vegetables like artichokes, beets, and potatoes. Afraid of the old pressure cookers that sounded like they were about to explode? There are now automatic pressure cookers, like the Instant Pot, that manage the time and pressure for you.

Note: Just recently I saw that it was under half an hour until dinner time and we had nothing cooked or thawed. I put some frozen chicken, frozen vegetables, dried navy beans, and natural bullion in the pressure cooker. We had an on-time dinner of delicious navy bean soup made from scratch.

MICROPLANE

Our recipes rely heavily on culinary spices and herbs. They are documented to improve liver function through these chemical constituents and from their interactions with the taste buds. The problem with many of them is that fresh is best, but the shelf life is short. So, get yourself a microplane and store your fresh spices in the freezer. When you need some fresh ginger, or turmeric, take the frozen version out, grate as much as you need, and return the rest to the freezer.

LET'S GO SHOPPING!

The secret to breezing through your Reset is planning. Thankfully, the shopping is already planned for you. If you plan to follow the menu plan, there are shopping lists compiled in advance. These involve one trip per week, since produce will not last much longer. Visit Chapter 5 for the shopping lists for each week.

Additionally, it works best to get your protein powder and resistant starch in advance. Since they are nonperishable and essential for the Reset program, obtain the full supply of 56 servings per person, or 112 servings per couple. Here is what to look for.

SHAKE INGREDIENTS

The Reset program provides optimal protein on a low-fuel diet. Pea-derived, plant-based protein powder is the best way to get the optimal protein. The better versions of it taste great. *Pea protein* lets you avoid the most common reactive foods, and it keeps your body in an alkaline state.

Avoid protein powders with added refined sugar, allergens, or synthetic flavors. For those who are not dairy intolerant, there are other options, including nonfat unsweetened Greek or Icelandic yogurt. The drawback with whey, soy, or egg protein is that these are more anabolic, which means they may help you bulk up but may not help you get lean.

The second most critical shake ingredient is *resistant starch*. This is helpful because it aids the liver in breaking down triglycerides and speeds the rate of converting adipose tissue into energy. Each shake should contain at least 10 grams of RS per serving. The best way to get RS is to use a protein powder that includes it, like the original Reset Shake (see page 119). Next-best options are blended RS supplements with no added sugar, or making a blend at home with RS2 pea starch, green banana flour, and unmodified potato starch.

STEP 4—TRACK YOUR PROGRESS

Did you take the metabolism quiz on page 5? If not, please go back and do so now. Make note of your score, as you'll recheck it as you go through the Reset. You might be amazed at how quickly it improves.

DITCH THE SCALE

Is it worth the weight? For years, many of us, including myself, have used the number on the scale as a barometer of our value and self-worth. Not only is this counterproductive for one's mental health, but it turns out that weight is not even the best way to track one's health.

WEIGHT LOSS OR WAIST LOSS?

So, trade your scale for a tape measure. It is time to forget about your weight. Body weight does not take into account body composition (body fat). Weight and weight-based markers like BMI are no longer considered valid for determining body size. In fact, a large recent study looked at all the published research on various measurements, including BMI, and found that height-to-waist ratio (HtWR) is a more accurate predictor of disease risk and longevity.[1] It is also much simpler to measure and track.

The ideal HtWR is between 0.4 and 0.5; this is your height divided by your waist circumference. Quite simply, your waist measurement should be at least half your height. Gender differences are minimal. Readings above 0.5 correlate with greater rates of chronic disease and premature death.

What should your waist circumference be? If you know your height, take a peek at the graph that follows. It shows the upper limit, lower limit, and median of healthy HtWR scores. Risks are higher when you are above the upper limit and are lowest at the median. If you are over the upper limit, use it for your first target. If you are slightly below the upper limit, work to move toward the median score.

If you are still watching the scale, here are some numbers to help you relate. For most adults, $\frac{1}{2}$ inch around the waist equals about 3 to 4 pounds of weight. It is not uncommon to see waist loss of several inches during the four-week Reset. This is unique because typical diets cause dramatic weight loss in the first week, but have little if any effect on waist size. We now know that the dramatic initial "weight loss" is just fluid loss and it comes right back. The four-week Reset causes more pronounced waist loss. Even if you have 3 to 4 inches to lose, you find yourself all the way back on track by the end of the four weeks.

HOW TO MEASURE YOUR WAIST

Here are a few tips to help you get an accurate waist measurement. First, get a paper or cloth tape measure. Plan to measure daily, first thing in the morning—after using the bathroom and before eating or drinking

HEIGHT	HEALTHY LIMITS FOR WAIST CIRCUMFERENCE		
	Lower	Median	Upper
4'10"	23.2	26.1	29
4'11"	23.6	26.5	29.5
5'0"	24	27	30
5'1"	24.4	27.5	30.5
5'2"	24.8	27.9	31
5'3"	25.2	28.4	31.5
5'4"	25.6	28.8	32
5'5"	26	29.3	32.5
5'6"	26.4	29.7	33
5'7"	26.8	30.2	33.5
5'8"	27.2	30.6	34
5'9"	27.7	31.1	34.5
5'10"	28	31.5	35
5'11"	28.4	32	35.5
6'0"	28.8	32.4	36
6'1"	29.2	32.9	36.5
6'2"	29.6	33.3	37
6'3"	30	33.8	37.5
6'4"	30.4	34.2	38
6'5"	30.8	34.7	38.5
6'6"	31.2	35.1	39

anything. There are normal fluctuations in the measurement, but checking more often helps you see the trend. Do not be alarmed when one day's measurement is higher or lower than the last.

To take the reading, breathe out and relax your abdominal muscles completely. It may feel scary to let it all out but remember that we want to be able to see progress; the more you may not like your "before" readings, the easier it is to get good "after" readings, okay? Now, measure around your waistline in line with your belly button, with the measuring tape parallel to the ground. Log your reading in your Reset journal.

OPTIONAL METRICS

The metabolism quiz score and your waist circumference are the most critical measures to keep an eye on, and you can do fine by just regularly checking those. But here are a few more optional markers that you may consider.

BODY FAT PERCENTAGE

The most accurate way to know how much adipose tissue you have is simply by measuring it. Body-fat measurements accurately predict the accumulation of liver fat, the risk of heart disease, and arterial stiffness.[2]

There are a few ways to calculate body fat, each with various advantages and disadvantages. Of all the methods available, I encourage readers to have a home bioelectrical impedance device and track it weekly. Good units can be found for $30 to $55 and are simple to use. They estimate body fat by measuring how well your body conducts a harmless electric current. Most devices are handheld and measure the current passing from one hand to another. The next most common types are integrated into a scale and they measure the current from one foot to another. The basic idea is that fat blocks the current more than lean tissue does. The better meters for home use are within 3 to 5 percent accuracy when you use them as directed. This level of accuracy is more than close enough to be useful and, even if they are off slightly, they are still accurate to track your day-to-day changes. You can also find scales with built-in body-fat testers for roughly the cost of a typical scale. If you already have a good scale, handheld units are also available. Any unit from a major manufacturer like Omron, Tanita, or Nokia will be effective.

Other body-fat measuring devices include calipers, immersion pods, and X-ray machines. If you regularly work with a trainer who is skilled in using calipers, they are a reasonable option. Other devices can be useful, but are less cost-effective for measuring on a weekly basis. Whereas any of the methods described will give consistent readings, you should stick with one method because you will not likely see the same readings when you go from one device to another.

As for the measurements themselves, any woman over 30 percent body fat, or a man over 25 percent body fat, is at risk for the complications of adiposity. It seems that some people are more sensitive to fat than others. If you are slightly below these targets, yet have abnormal levels of cholesterol, blood sugar, or blood pressure, your body may be less fat tolerant. Populations with the lowest rates of modern disease tend to be quite lean, with women averaging between 20 to 25 percent body fat and men at 13 to 20 percent body fat.

MORNING GLUCOSE

One of the most important parts of an annual blood panel can be easily measured at home for under $2 per reading. Most pharmacies have blood glucose meters for $15 to $30 and the strips cost about $1 each.

When the liver becomes less able to manage fuel, more fuel often stays in the bloodstream. This extra fuel is measurable by seeing how much glucose is in circulation before eating. When you sleep at night, you are not eating and your liver is almost solely in charge of keeping enough glucose in your bloodstream. When your liver gets clogged, however, it makes too much glucose in an attempt to get rid of the extra fuel.

If your liver is healthy, your morning fasting blood sugar should be between 70 and 85. If you are above 99, you are considered at risk for diabetes. You may be interested to see how dramatically this number can change during the course of the four-week Reset. In our clinic, we have seen many people go from readings of over 200—well in the diabetic range—to readings in the low 90s.

RESTING HEART RATE

Your resting heart rate is how often your heart beats each minute. This is a good gauge of how efficiently your cardiovascular system is working. Your liver filters your entire blood supply every second of the day. The more clogged it is, the harder your heart and blood vessels need to work. This is one of the reasons that fatty liver causes higher risks for high blood pressure and heart disease.

A 2013 study showed that the best resting heart rate was 50 beats per minute or under. For every 10 beats per minute, over 50, there was a 16 percent annual increase risk of death. A resting heart rate over 90 corresponded with a near doubling of the death risk.[3]

To measure your resting heart rate (RHR), do so first thing in the morning, before eating or consuming caffeine. Use your index and middle finger and feel your heart rate on your neck or opposite wrist, counting for a full minute. Many see their RHR decrease by 8 to 14 beats per minute over the course of their Reset.

URINARY KETONES

Ketone testing is not necessary, but may be helpful if you experience intense hunger or food cravings. The goal of the Reset is not to go deep into ketosis, but if you reduce your fuel enough, you will likely have a mild elevation of ketones, which often suppresses hunger. Urinary ketone test strips do not use uniform units, but expect them to be in mild to moderate ketosis. If you are not at least in mild ketosis, double-check your fuel intake, as you may be taking in more than is best for you. Most people find that after their first few days, hunger and food cravings drop off. They also notice a heightened sense of mental clarity and often better well-being. Physical energy may be lower, which is why it is essential to reduce exercise to the recommended micro workouts.

STEP 5—GET A SUPPORT TEAM

Talk to your friends and family about your plan. Share with them a few of the reasons you discovered during your journaling exercise.

FAMILY, SPOUSE, PARTNER, CHILDREN, ROOMMATES

Talk to everyone who shares meals with you before you start. Do it in a big group or one-on-one session. Let them know you would like their help in choosing recipes, and that they will not be limited to their portion sizes. In turn, give the following gentle requests for the next four weeks:

1. Keep unplanned snacks and junk food away from the house and away from you.

2. Any restaurant chosen must have light and healthy options.

3. You will need to be asleep at a time that will give you eight hours of sleep before your morning duties. Others can stay up as late as they like, but they have to be quiet.

COWORKERS

Invite others to participate and choose a date in advance. Try something like: "Hey, I'm doing a Reset diet starting the first of this coming month. Who would like to do it with me?" Most office cultures love the idea of a group effort. You can even make it a competition between teams—completion based on consistency, not on outcome. Owing to different genes, gender, and on how far someone has to go, some people will lose inches much faster than others.

If coworkers bring snacks or you normally share meals, let them know that for four weeks starting on x date, you'll be bringing your own shakes in place of lunch and will be avoiding snacks besides healthy produce. They can do what they wish, but let them know ahead of time that you have a plan. They may still offer you other food, but if you let them know in advance, it will take less of your effort to dissuade their well-intentioned offers.

ACCOUNTABILITY PARTNER

Find a friend who would also like to do a Metabolism Reset. Meet up for daily (short) walks and share notes on your experience and progress. Talk through any stumbling blocks that come up and share the solutions that work for you. If no one in your area comes to mind, consider social media.

There is an instant community ready to connect with you and support you at metabolismresetdietbook.com. Post a question, find a new recipe, and see some inspirational stories to keep you moving forward. Indeed, look for me and say Hi. I check in often.

REVIEW AND PREPARATION CHECKLIST

- ☐ Selected start date for the reset
- ☐ Created Reset journal
- ☐ Recorded journal entries about reasons for the reset
- ☐ Measured and recorded first entry of waist log
- ☐ Measured morning heart rate and recorded first entry in heart rate log
- ☐ Found an accountability partner(s)
- ☐ Notified spouse and kids of Reset guidelines
- ☐ Bought and ordered program staples
- ☐ Purchased first week's perishables

It looks like you are ready for a whole new chapter in your life. In the next chapter of this book, you will learn the exact foods and amounts that will take you there. Let's do it!

chapter five

Food for the Metabolism Reset

Remember, food is the medicine that will heal your liver so that you can reset your metabolism. Here is where you will get the exact prescriptions.

Since humans are omnivores, your body is able to thrive on a broad variety of foods. You do not need to be paleo or vegan to have a healthy liver, but if you are, you can still do fine on this Reset. You also will not need to go out of your way to find exotic ingredients or invest more than you already do in groceries. All the recipes can be made with simple ingredients that you can find in any grocery store.

The Metabolism Reset is set up to keep the menu simple. Studies have shown that people are more successful making large changes in their lives that are simple rather than smaller changes that are more complicated. Successful participants typically look at this chapter and Chapter 7 with the recipes before starting the program. So, before diving in, get a good grasp of how the Reset works and plan a start date.

Each day's menu has three elements:

- Two shakes: one for breakfast and another for lunch
- One meal for dinner
- Unlimited snacks whenever you need them

The most significant change people typically notice is the shift to having a shake for lunch. Many already have a shake or something else that's light for breakfast, and dinner is not all that different from what is often typical. You can expect to get used to this new routine within the first week. Give yourself the first several days to adjust, and do not worry if it feels odd at the beginning. Soon, you will likely find yourself appreciating the improved mental clarity. The other benefit that many people notice early on is that they do not need to spend as much time on food preparation as usual.

Let's start by learning how to make your shakes!

THE BREAKFAST SHAKE

Mix and drink your first shake within an hour of waking up. Once you blend the ingredients, the taste and texture are good for several hours.

It can work to make a double batch of your shake in the morning and that way you'll have lunch already taken care of. If you do make your lunch shake in advance, it may separate during the morning hours, in which case just give it a quick stir or two. However, it usually does not work well to make the breakfast shake the night before.

If you do get hungry easily, drink your shake more slowly. Try drinking your shake through a straw—it can cause you to consume it over a longer period of time and allow your body more of a chance to turn off any sensations of hunger. Look for straws made of glass or stainless steel, and choose those that are wider than typical straws, since the consistency of shakes is thicker than that of other beverages.

HOW TO MAKE A RESET SHAKE

Make flavor your highest priority. Convenience is also important, but all the ingredients have long shelf lives and do not require elaborate preparation. I cannot overemphasize this point: you must love the way your shake tastes, and it is worth taking the time to get it right.

First, browse through the recipes in Chapter 7 and find five that catch your eye. Maybe you will start with something like Frozen Hot "Cocoa" (page 123), the Classic Green Smoothie (page 124), or Carrot Spice Cake (page 127). Because a small number of ingredients are used in numerous shake recipes, you can shop for these items and still have everything you need to make them all. Once you have those first few recipes working well for you, mix and match by using the Shake Assembly Guide below.

BLENDER

You'll need a blender to make your shakes. Any kind can work well for all these recipes. Some ingredients will have the best texture when a high-powered appliance is used—for example, Blendtec, Vitamix, NutriBullet, and Ninja blender.

SHAKE ASSEMBLY GUIDE

There are a few shake ingredients worth covering in a bit of detail ahead of time, including protein, resistant starch, seeds, and natural flavorings, plus some optional superfoods.

PROTEIN

For best results on your reset, please choose a protein source that has no artificial ingredients, no common allergens, no refined sugar, and at least 20 grams of protein per serving. The best options are also pH neutral.

In the Metabolism Reset clinical trials, we use a custom meal replacement that utilizes high-grade pea protein isolate.

Dairy-based proteins such as whey or casein are best avoided since they may slow thyroid function due to their iodine content. Beef-based protein sources can be good for day-to-day use but are best avoided during the Reset since they can contribute to the acid load on the kidneys and impair detoxification. Rice-based protein is best avoided since it lacks many essential amino acids needed for optimal liver function.

If you choose to make your own shake, the top choice protein option is:

- Pea protein powder (1 serving)

The second choice protein option is:

- Blended vegetable protein powder (1 serving)

Other protein options:

- Hydro beef protein powder (1 serving)
- Liquid egg whites (1 cup); do not use raw egg whites since they are unpasteurized and carry the risk of salmonella, and they may deplete biotin
- Soy protein powder (1 serving)

RESISTANT STARCH (RS)

Numerous studies show that the short-term benefits of RS require doses of 15,000–25,000 mg daily. In the Metabolism Reset Diet clinical trials, we use the Original Reset Shake, which includes 12,000 mg of RS per serving and uses two servings daily for a total of 24,000 mg of RS.

If you wish to make your own shake, you can also use a commercial resistant starch blend such as RS Complete. Commercial RS blends have no taste and can help supply the full amount of RS needed for the Metabolism Reset. Do consider their ingredients since some people avoid certain food sources used in their manufacture.

There are also many foods that are rich sources of RS. For long-term use, all of the foods rich in RS are good to include in the diet and are highly recommended. For the Metabolism Reset Diet, foods can also be used in shakes, but it may not be possible to achieve the 15,000–20,000 mg of RS that was used in most clinical trials without exceeding the recommended fuel content of the shake. Please also consider the effect that food sources of RS may have on the taste and texture of the shake.

Food sources of RS:

- Green banana flour ($\frac{1}{4}$ cup). Amount of RS per serving: 3,000–6,000 mg
- Frozen organic ripe banana with peel ($\frac{1}{2}$). Amount of RS per serving: 2,000–4,000 mg
- White beans ($\frac{1}{4}$ cup), either navy, great northern, or cannellini. Amount of RS per serving: 1,500–2,000 mg
- Aquafaba ($\frac{1}{2}$ cup). Amount of RS per serving: 1,200–1,800 mg

FROZEN BANANAS

Several recipes call for frozen bananas because they add rich flavor and can provide some RS. You can also use banana peels! They contain more resistant starch, potassium, magnesium, and more vitamin B_6 than the fruit itself.

If you do plan to use the peels, organic bananas are mandatory and work better when they are ripe. If you are not using the peels, use unripe bananas. Those with some green on the skin will have more resistant starch and will be digested more slowly.

Cut the peeled bananas into quarters, and freeze in a glass storage container. To use bananas with the peel, trim off the tip and stem, then cut into quarters and freeze in a glass storage container. Note: The peel works better in smoothies when you use a high-powered blender. It's worth trying a smoothie or two with the peel, if you have not done so. There is no significant taste impact, but it does provide a richer texture.

RS TIPS

The RS foods and seeds are easy additions because they do not have much flavor of their own. If your diet has been low in fiber for some time, such as a paleo diet, you may want to start with a quarter to half the specified amount of RS. You still have the flora to digest it, but they are fewer in number at first. Once you have had even small amounts of RS foods for a few weeks, you can begin having them in unrestricted quantities.

SEEDS

Use ¹/₂ to 1 tablespoon of any of the following:

- Sunflower seeds
- Flax seeds
- Chia seeds
- Hemp seeds
- Sesame seeds

NATURAL FLAVORINGS

Use unlimited quantities of any of the following:

- Stevia
- Lo han fruit extract
- Xylitol
- Cinnamon
- Ginger
- Natural extracts (vanilla, almond, etc.)
- Food-grade essential oils (lemon, wild orange, peppermint)

SWEETENERS

Most of the recipes work better with a sweetener. I recommend stevia, lo han, or xylitol. These are safe and have no significant effect on cravings or blood sugar levels. Note that xylitol can act as a laxative when used in high dosages. Some people may notice this effect at lower doses more than others but most people do fine with a few teaspoons of it at a time.

The differences between stevia and lo han come down to personal taste preferences. If you have not already done so, please try both to see what you prefer. The sweeteners can also vary significantly from brand to brand. If you do not like the first brand, try a few more and remember which one works best for you.

Because of these variations in products and personal preferences, the recipes do not specify amounts of sweetener. Typical amounts of stevia that people prefer can range a lot. Some like a few drops, others use a few droppers full. Lo han is similar. With either, it is better to start with a few drops and work up gradually. The concentration of sweetness in xylitol is close to that of table sugar; most people will do best using a few teaspoons or tablespoons for a shake.

Many other natural sweeteners still have a substantial burden of fuel and are best avoided in the Reset shakes. These include coconut sugar, sucanat, turbinado sugar, agave nectar, honey, molasses, date sugar, and brown rice syrup.

AQUAFABA

A large amount of the enjoyment of shakes has as much to do with the texture as it does with the flavor. This is why most shake recipes use milk or some kind of a milk substitute. The drawback of milk and milk substitutes is that they are high in fuel and low in protein. That is why I use aquafaba as a thickener and extra source of RS in the recipes.

The name *aquafaba* means "water from beans" and that's really all it is. It has no taste of its own, but it makes a wonderful texture in shakes. I'm not the first to sing its praises—it is a great ingredient for lots of recipes. If you choose to leave it out, the shakes will work fine, but just be sure to supply enough RS from another source.

The main two ways to get aquafaba are to just take the liquid from canned beans or to make your own. Be sure the cans are BPA free, with no ingredients besides the beans and water. If the beans are salted or lightly salted, it will work, but unsalted will work best. Drain the liquid from a can of chickpeas or white beans, then use the liquid in a shake and store the beans in the refrigerator for use within the next 48 hours.

If cooking the beans, place 1 pound of dried chickpeas (approximately 2 cups) in a large fine-mesh colander. Pick through the beans and discard any that are not mature. Rinse well for 2 minutes, then pour the chickpeas into a large bowl and cover with 5 cups water. Cover and let sit for 12 hours or overnight. Then transfer the chickpeas and liquid to a saucepan, add water if need be so that chickpeas are covered by at least 1 inch, and bring to a boil. Reduce the heat and simmer until the chickpeas are soft, anywhere from 40 minutes to 1 hour. If the water level goes below the surface of the beans, you may need to add water. Drain the chickpeas. The resulting liquid should be about the same thickness as the aquafaba from a can of chickpeas. If it seems too thin, simmer a bit longer in the saucepan until the desired consistency is reached. The aquafaba liquid can be stored, covered, in the refrigerator for up to 5 days.

If aquafaba is not an option and you do want a texturizer, frozen bananas also do the job. Another option is unsweetened flax milk. This is the only milk substitute that has essential fats and is low in fuel. However, do not use it in addition to aquafaba. Also, do not use cow's milk, almond milk, coconut milk, rice milk, or other milk substitutes.

OPTIONAL SUPERFOODS

- Greens (1 cup), such as spinach, kale, chard
- Milk thistle seeds (1 tablespoon)
- Spirulina (1 teaspoon)
- MCT (1 teaspoon)
- Maca (1 teaspoon)
- Roasted carob powder (1 teaspoon)
- Mesquite powder (1 teaspoon)
- Cordyceps powder (1 teaspoon)

OPTIONAL SHAKE FRUIT

Use only for shakes, and no more than $1/2$ fruit or less per breakfast or lunch serving.

- Dark cherries
- Strawberries
- Oranges
- Bananas
- Peaches

- Plums
- Raspberries
- Blueberries
- Kiwi
- Papaya

- Pomegranates
- Apples

- Raisins (organic)
- Blackberries

Maybe you are a chef who can eyeball ingredients and automatically create a masterpiece. If not, start with some of the shake recipes in Chapter 7. Then, when you've gotten accustomed to making the shakes, you can fashion your own just by choosing one of each of the items from the protein, resistant starch, and seed listings and then add any of the optional flavors and superfoods.

However you make your shake, you may be pleasantly surprised to find that you come to like them increasingly as you go. The more time you spend avoiding processed foods with exaggerated flavors, the more your taste buds will physically change. You will come to enjoy the rich and complex flavors of natural foods more than ever. When you eat less, your appetite improves, and the more often you taste a certain flavor when you are truly hungry, the more you will come to like it.

MID-MORNING SNACKS

Snacks are there if you need them, but they are not mandatory. You may find that they seem essential the first few days, then you may be indifferent to them.

If you do find yourself hungry, "unlimited foods" means a lot more than celery sticks. You have tons of great options, such as Carrot Fries (page 197), Fresh Spring Gazpacho (page 202), or Savory Eggplant Boats (page 204). You can find recipes like these and more in the "Unlimited Recipes" section of Chapter 8.

Along with these recipes, you can make your own snacks with any combination of the following, raw or cooked, with any of the unlimited seasonings.

Unlimited veggies are:

- Alfalfa sprouts
- Arugula
- Artichokes (whole)

- Artichoke hearts
- Asparagus
- Bamboo shoots

- Bean sprouts
- Bok choy and baby bok choy
- Broccoli
- Brussels sprouts
- Butter lettuce
- Cabbage
- Carrots
- Cauliflower
- Celery
- Celery root
- Chicory greens
- Collard greens
- Crookneck squash
- Cucumbers
- Daikon
- Eggplant
- Endive
- Escarole
- Fennel
- Garlic
- Green beans
- Green leaf lettuce
- Green onions/Scallions
- Green peppers
- Jicama
- Kale
- Kohlrabi
- Leaf lettuce
- Leeks
- Lemon juice
- Lime juice
- Mushrooms
- Okra
- Onions
- Pea pods
- Pumpkin
- Radicchio
- Radishes
- Red leaf lettuce
- Red peppers
- Romaine lettuce
- Rutabaga
- Snow peas
- Spaghetti squash
- Spinach
- Summer squash
- Swiss chard
- Tomatoes
- Tomatillos
- Turnip greens
- Water chestnuts
- Watercress
- Zucchini

Some of these are easy grab-and-go foods, like baby carrots, yet with a little planning and preparation, a snack can be as filling and elaborate as homemade tomato sauce with mushrooms served over spaghetti squash and zucchini noodles.

LUNCH

Lunch is super-easy because you have already made it. Of course, you can make a brand-new shake, but it is so handy to just make a double batch in the morning.

Plan to have your lunch shake within four to six hours of your breakfast shake. Since this is a shake, and it can be premade, there is no reason to delay it any longer than this. The goal is to have a solid dose of protein three times daily to supply your liver with the amino acids necessary for detoxification, and to keep your body from breaking down your muscles.

Once you have breakfast figured out, lunch is so simple because all the same recommendations apply. In the morning, you can make your lunch shake in a nonplastic bottle and take it along with you, or you can make up something fresh when the moment arises.

Even when you have a shake for lunch, notice how you feel when you still take the time to focus on eating. Rather than gulping it down while you are working on a project, see how you feel when you make lunch an event. Go to a new location, ideally outdoors. Put your phone away and focus on your meal, allowing at least 15 to 20 minutes to complete it. It turns out that much of hunger is psychological. When you do not make a meal your top mental focus, it will not satisfy you as much. It takes some time and focus for your brain to register the fact that you just had a meal.

If you occasionally have a business or social gathering for lunch, you can flip lunch and dinner. Have a shake for dinner and follow your meal guidelines for lunch. Up to twice per week works as a harmless variation.

MID-AFTERNOON SNACKS

Just like mid-morning snacks, these are optional and may become less important to you after your first few days on the Reset. Since you may be on the go at this time, plan what you will bring with you the day before and have it ready.

DINNER

Not only do you still get to eat dinner, you get to eat well. I was so happy to see that the Reset could be just as effective with a solid meal each day. This meal makes people feel fuller and sleep better. It also makes it easier to stick with the program and get the total benefits.

Like your other meals, dinner can be elaborate and gourmet or be a quick production from meal-assembly and batch-cooking techniques. Your Reset calendar will walk you through the rhythm of shopping and preparation, so that your dinners will be a welcome bookend to your day.

Visit Chapter 8 for tons of great recipe ideas, like Shepherd's Pie (page 166), Vegan Pumpkin Risotto (page 170), Fall Vegetable Beef Roast (page 171), and many more. Once you get the hang of the basic recipes, you can also make your own favorites using this Dinner Assembly Guide.

DINNER ASSEMBLY GUIDE

PROTEIN

You have lots of options, whether on a vegan, vegetarian, or paleo diet. As much as possible, try to use a variety of protein foods from one day to the next. The protein options are a 4- to 6-ounce serving of any one of the following foods:

- Chicken
- Whitefish
- Cottage cheese ($^1/_2$ cup)
- Lean grass-fed beef
- Mussels and oysters
- Shrimp

- Pork tenderloin
- Salmon
- Tempeh
- Tofu
- Turkey
- Sardines in water

You can also use the following protein sources for variety. Please note that it is not practical to get the full 30+ grams from them alone. These are options to be used in conjunction with other foods from the primary list.

- Edamame
- Nutritional yeast (folic acid-free)
- Spirulina
- ²/₃ cup yogurt (fat-free, high protein)

RESISTANT STARCH

Each dinner includes a food with resistant starch in order to reach the day's target intake. Along with RS, your food will supply a full spectrum of fibers so that you maintain a diverse and healthy flora. Dinner RS sources include rice, arrowroot, quinoa, and gluten-free pasta, along with:

High-starch veggies (1 cup)
- Boiled potatoes
- Sweet potato/yam
- Plantain
- Peas

Legumes, cooked (³/₄ cup)
- Lentils
- Chickpeas
- Navy beans
- Great northern beans
- Black beans
- Lotus seeds
- White beans
- Split peas
- Kidney beans

Intact whole grains, cooked (³/₄ cup)
- Buckwheat
- Oat groats
- Pearl barley

NUTRIENT-RICH VEGGIES

High-nutrient, low-fuel veggies will make up the majority of your dinner's volume. All of the veggies listed here are good, but they also include some of the best-documented liver helpers on a regular basis, like broccoli, cauliflower, cabbage, carrots, garlic, parsnips, and parsley.

- Artichokes
- Arugula
- Asparagus
- Beets and beet greens

- Bell peppers (red, green)
- Bok choy
- Broccoli
- Broccoli rabe
- Broccolini
- Brussels sprouts
- Cabbage
- Carrots
- Cauliflower
- Celery
- Collard greens
- Cucumbers
- Dandelion greens
- Eggplant
- Endive
- Escarole
- Fennel
- Green beans
- Green onions (scallions)
- Jicama
- Kale
- Leeks
- Mixed greens
- Mushrooms
- Mustard greens
- Okra
- Peppers
- Pumpkin
- Radicchio
- Radishes
- Romaine lettuce
- Shallots
- Snow peas
- Spaghetti squash
- Spinach
- Sprouts (all varieties)
- Summer squash
- Swiss chard
- Tomatoes (BPA-free cans)
- Turnip greens
- Watercress
- Wax beans

GOOD FATS

For fats, use 1 to 2 teaspoons of cooking oil or 1 to 2 tablespoons of nuts and seeds with your dinner. Since the healthiest oils are not always the most heat stable, follow the cooking guidelines in Chapter 8 and add oils at the final stages of cooking.

Best oils:
- Extra-virgin olive oil (EVOO)[1,2]
- Sesame oil[3] (or toasted sesame oil)
- Walnut oil[4]
- Avocado oil

Best nuts and seeds:

- Almonds
- Flax seeds
- Macadamia nuts
- Pecans
- Pistachios
- Sunflower seeds
- Walnuts

FLAVORINGS AND SEASONINGS

The right mix of herbs and seasonings will make your meals delicious, but they also serve an important role of their own. The sampling listed here will contribute to your Reset success but isn't an exhaustive list. If you follow the book's recipes, you will get a good variety of them and may learn some new favorites. If you are using the Dinner Assembly Guide to make your own meals, please remember to include them in your meals. When shopping for them, buy small quantities and store them in the freezer. Once you open them, the flavors tend to oxidize and degrade at room temperature even after just a few weeks.

Each week's shopping list will include herbs and condiments needed for that week's meals. Do not feel the need to rush out and buy them all right now.

Culinary herbs and spices:

- Asafetida
- Basil
- Black pepper
- Cardamom
- Chives
- Coriander
- Cumin
- Fennel
- Galangal
- Garlic
- Ginger
- Lemongrass
- Mint
- Nutmeg
- Oregano
- Paprika
- Rosemary
- Tarragon
- Thyme
- Turmeric

Optional condiments:

- Vinegars
- Hot sauce (sugar-free)
- Mustard (organic)
- Iodine-free sea salt ($^{1}/_{2}$ tsp per day max)
- Non-GMO tamari (organic)
- Thai fish sauce
- Miso
- Nutritional yeast
- Chicken and vegetable stock
- Coconut aminos

Now that you know the building blocks of your shakes and meals, you are welcome to make them based on what you like and what you have on hand. To make it easy, I have included suggested meals and shakes for each day of the entire program at the end of this chapter. If you want even more help, you can get shopping lists, recipe videos, and buyer's guides on the website metabolismresetdietbook.com.

BEVERAGES

What should you drink during your Reset? Focus on purified water. Believe it or not, when you drink your eight scheduled glasses of water, you will probably start to feel thirstier. When you are even a few percent below your fluid needs, it blocks you from feeling thirsty.

Mineral water is also an option when you would like some variety. Naturally carbonated mineral waters such as Perrier, San Pellegrino, or Gerolsteiner are tasty and also rich sources of magnesium and calcium. They are a harmless way to work in some variety to your meals. Try adding a squeeze of lime and a drop of wild orange oil in a large bottle.

In addition to water, there are these options.

NATURALLY CAFFEINE-FREE HERBAL TEAS

Many enjoy the ritual of a hot beverage in the morning or when doing mental work. If you like a rich, roasted flavor, try rooibos (pronounced ROY-boss). It is a naturally caffeine-free plant rich in flavors and health-promoting polyphenols. Other similar-tasting options include beverages made from toasted chicory, toasted dandelion root, and clearing nut. If you miss coffee, try products like Raja's Cup or the Teeccino line.

All other herbal teas can also be used freely. Lemon balm is great for mental alertness, peppermint can ease bloating or cramping, chamomile is nice to unwind with in the evenings.

ALCOHOL

Avoid all sources of alcohol during the Reset. The goal of the Reset diet is to heal the liver and make it able again to move fuel out of fat cells. Alcohol places a high demand on the liver's glycogen supply, which is already depleted in many who are overweight. It also forms the carcinogenic by-product called acetaldehyde, which places further demands on your liver.

CAFFEINE

Avoid all sources of caffeine during the Reset. This includes coffee, black tea, and green tea. Decaffeinated organic tea and organic coffee can be used as long as they are decaffeinated by the CO_2 process for tea or the Swiss water process for coffee. Other decaffeination processes are less effective, leaving as much as 30 mg of caffeine per serving, and they can leave solvent residues in the finished product.

Caffeine forces the liver to empty its glycogen stores, which is a big problem during the Reset. Many people who avoid sugar use caffeine without realizing that they both create a temporary spike in blood sugar, with all the negative consequences that go along with it. The other problem with caffeine is that it is one of the strongest activators of phase 1 liver pathways. Most with adiposity need more phase 2 activity relative to their phase 1 (see Chapter 3.)

After the Reset is over, a few servings of organic coffee and tea without creamer, butter, or sweeteners are harmless for most people and may even have some health benefits.

JUICES

During the Reset, you are welcome to make smoothies from the unlimited foods. Apart from that, avoid all juices, smoothies, and shakes besides those in the program. Even healthy foods make your liver work. The Reset relies on giving it enough downtime to rest and repair.

SODAS

Avoid all sodas during the Reset, even diet sodas. Regular sodas are the single worst food in terms of giving you empty calories without filling you up. Numerous studies have shown that soda has no impact on hunger. For example, if someone ingests 200 calories from soda in the morning, the individual will eat just about as much food throughout the rest of the day as he or she would have otherwise. Diet sodas, even natural ones, may increase appetite. Typical diet sodas also contain many synthetic ingredients and unhealthy additives.

The more important your recovery is to you, the more worthwhile it is to stick to the exact recipes and guidelines. For questions about special times like eating out and traveling, visit Chapter 10.

As important as food is, your lifestyle can still make or break your Reset efforts. In the next chapter, you will get the detailed plan for exercise, sleep, and calming your mind. These are all essential steps to take so that your results can last.

A MEAL PLAN FOR THE RESET

Here is a suggested complete menu for the four-week Reset. If you choose to follow it, you will have the benefit of a new dinner each night, a new shake each day, shopping lists for each week, and specific ideas for unlimited foods each day. You also have the option of using the Dinner Assembly Guide and the Shake Assembly Guide (see pages 72 and 63) to fill in some days, as well as the choice of following the traveling suggestions in Chapter 10 for days when you are on the road.

With these suggested recipes and menus, the default recommendation is to make your shakes in one session each morning. If your blender has room, double the recipe and make it all at once. If not, just keep the ingredients out and make a second batch right after finishing the first. Refrigerate the lunch portion in a glass or steel container or pack it with you in a small cooler if you will be away from home for lunch. Please note that these suggestions are exactly that: suggestions. If you do not feel a need for them on a given day, feel free to skip them. Most people are less hungry after the first few days of the Reset. When shopping for dried goods pantry items, first check to see if you have ingredients left over from previous weeks.

Also, please note that some listings do not refer to recipes in the book; these are, instead, suggestions for types of produce that lend themselves to be handy snacks. The shopping lists can also be downloaded in printer-friendly form at metabolismresetdietbook.com.

WEEK 1 SHOPPING LIST

PRODUCE

- ☐ Strawberries (organic), 1 pint
- ☐ Navel oranges (organic), 1 package
- ☐ Fresh spinach, 2 bags
- ☐ Bananas, 6 medium
- ☐ Papaya, 1 medium
- ☐ Fresh ginger, 3 pieces
- ☐ Lemons, 5
- ☐ Carrots or baby carrots, 10 to 14 (about ½ pound)
- ☐ Garlic, 2 heads and 6 cloves
- ☐ Shallot, 1 medium
- ☐ White onion, 1 large
- ☐ Celery, 7 stalks
- ☐ Zucchini, 1 medium
- ☐ Cauliflower, 1 head
- ☐ Yellow onions, 4 medium
- ☐ Sweet onion, 1 large
- ☐ Red potatoes, 4 to 5 medium
- ☐ Rutabaga (yellow turnip), 1 medium
- ☐ Cherry tomatoes, 2 pints
- ☐ Yellow potatoes, 3 medium
- ☐ Lettuce, 1 head
- ☐ Lime, 1
- ☐ Lemongrass, 2 stalks
- ☐ Thai chile, 1
- ☐ Fresh cilantro, 2 bunches

☐ Fresh chives, 1 bunch

☐ Orange bell peppers, roasted, 4 to 5

☐ Red, yellow, or orange bell peppers, 5

☐ Fresh tomatoes, 8 medium

☐ Fresh parsley, 2 bunches

☐ Fresh basil, 1 bunch

☐ Eggplant, 2 medium

☐ Shiitake mushrooms, 1 (16-ounce) package

☐ Cucumbers, 4 large

☐ Fresh tarragon, 1 bunch

☐ Fresh thyme, 1 bunch

☐ Avocado, 1 medium

MEATS/FISH

☐ Salmon fillet, 1 pound

☐ Ground turkey, $1\frac{1}{2}$ pounds

☐ Beef roast (organic), 2–3 pounds (boneless)

☐ Shrimp (wild-caught), 3 pounds

☐ Chicken breast (organic), 1 pound

BEVERAGES

☐ Vegetable juice cocktail or tomato puree (organic), 1 (16-ounce) bottle

☐ Tomato juice, 1 (15-ounce) can

FROZEN FOODS

None

BREAD/BAKERY

None

DAIRY

None

CANNED/JARRED GOODS

- ☐ Whole-grain Dijon mustard, 1 (4-ounce) can
- ☐ Tomato paste, 1 (6-ounce) can
- ☐ Beef broth (organic), 1 (32-ounce) container
- ☐ Vegetable or chicken stock (organic), 1 (32-ounce) container
- ☐ White beans, 2 (15-ounce) cans
- ☐ Chickpeas (garbanzo beans), 1 (15-ounce) can

- ☐ Coconut milk, light, 1 (15-ounce) can
- ☐ Capers, 1 (4-ounce) jar
- ☐ Fish sauce, Thai or Vietnamese 1 (8-ounce) bottle
- ☐ Apple cider vinegar, 1 (16-ounce) bottle
- ☐ Red wine vinegar, 1 (16-ounce) bottle
- ☐ Balsamic vinegar, 1 (16-ounce) bottle

DRIED GOODS/PANTRY ITEMS

- ☐ Sweetener, like stevia, lo han, xylitol powder, 1 (1-ounce) package
- ☐ Pea protein powder (or other protein base), 14 servings
- ☐ Vanilla extract, 1 (4-ounce) bottle
- ☐ Steel-cut or old-fashioned rolled oats (gluten-free), 1 (32-ounce) package
- ☐ Carob powder, toasted, 1/4 pound
- ☐ Chia seeds, 1/4 pound
- ☐ Dried turmeric, 1 (0.5-ounce or larger) container
- ☐ Ceylon cinnamon, 1 (0.5-ounce or larger) container
- ☐ Whole cloves, 1 (0.5-ounce or larger) jar
- ☐ Almonds, 1 (16-ounce) package
- ☐ Green banana flour, 1 (16-ounce) container

- ☐ Ground nutmeg, 1 (0.5-ounce or larger) container
- ☐ Brown rice, 1 (28-ounce) package
- ☐ Salt
- ☐ Black pepper, 1 (0.5-ounce or larger) container
- ☐ Avocado oil, (16-ounce) bottle
- ☐ Extra-virgin olive oil, (16-ounce) bottle
- ☐ Dried thyme, 1 (0.5-ounce or larger) jar
- ☐ Red pepper flakes, 1 (0.5-ounce or larger) container
- ☐ Dried parsley, 1 (1-ounce or larger) jar
- ☐ Paprika, 1 (0.5-ounce or larger) container
- ☐ Cayenne pepper, 1 (0.5-ounce or larger) container

	WEEK 1 MENUS	PAGE
DAY 1	**SHAKE** Strawberry Orange Sunrise	121
	DINNER 10-Minute Grilled Salmon Bowl	152
	UNLIMITED FOOD SUGGESTION Carrot Fries	197
DAY 2	**SHAKE** Roasted Strawberry Smoothie	122
	DINNER Shepherd's Pie	166
	UNLIMITED FOOD SUGGESTION Roasted Orange Pepper Soup	201
DAY 3	**SHAKE** Frozen Hot "Cocoa"	123
	DINNER Fall Vegetable Beef Roast	171
	UNLIMITED FOOD SUGGESTION Savory Eggplant Boats	204
DAY 4	**SHAKE** Classic Green Smoothie	124
	DINNER Spicy Shrimp and Beans	180
	UNLIMITED FOOD SUGGESTION Asian Broth	206
DAY 5	**SHAKE** Almond Crunch Oatmeal	125
	DINNER Egg-Free Niçoise Salad	193
	UNLIMITED FOOD SUGGESTION baby carrots	
DAY 6	**SHAKE** Papaya Ginger Mint	126
	DINNER Best Thai Chicken Coconut Soup	181
	UNLIMITED FOOD SUGGESTION Fresh Spring Gazpacho	202
DAY 7	**SHAKE** Carrot Spice Cake	127
	DINNER Baked Shrimp with Lemon and Chives	185
	UNLIMITED FOOD SUGGESTION Zesty Cucumber-Pepper Rainbow Salad	200

WEEK 2 SHOPPING LIST

PRODUCE

☐ Pomegranate, 1

☐ Fresh spinach,
     2 (8-ounce) bags

☐ Fresh rosemary, 1 bunch

☐ Granny Smith apple,
     1 medium

☐ Beets, 1 bunch

☐ Pineapple, 1

☐ Fresh coconut, 1

☐ Fresh mint, 1 bunch

☐ Green cabbage,
     1 medium head

☐ Sweet or yellow onions,
     4 medium

☐ Garlic, 6 medium heads

☐ Fresh basil, 3 bunches

☐ Carrots, 7 large

☐ Limes, 3

☐ Fresh ginger, 1 (3-inch) piece

☐ Broccoli, 1 head

☐ Red bell pepper, 1

☐ Green onions, 5

☐ Peanuts, 1 (8-ounce)
     package, shelled

☐ Fresh parsley, 1 bunch

☐ Baby potatoes, 1 pound

☐ Green beans, 1 pound

☐ Red onions, 3 medium

☐ Small red potatoes,
     1 pound

☐ Lettuce, 2 heads

☐ Fresh cilantro, 1 bunch

☐ Lemon, 1

☐ Zucchinis, 6 to 8 medium

☐ Tomatoes, 4 medium

☐ Celery, 6 stalks

☐ Shiitake mushrooms,
     2 (16-ounce) packages

☐ Lemongrass, 1 stalk

☐ Snow peas,
     1 (16-ounce) package

☐ Cauliflower florets,
     1 (16-ounce) package

☐ Fennel, 1 bulb

☐ Green beans, 1 pound

☐ Cherry tomatoes, 1 pint

MEATS/FISH

☐ Ground meat, 1 pound

☐ Alaskan salmon fillet
     (wild-caught), 1 pound

☐ Chicken breasts (organic),
  2 breasts, split
  (about 1½ pounds)

☐ Atlantic cod fillet
  (wild-caught), 1 pound

☐ Canned salmon (wild-caught),
  1 (15-ounce) can

☐ Chicken (organic), 1 pound

BEVERAGES

None

FROZEN FOODS

☐ Dark cherries, frozen,
  (16-ounce) package

BREAD/BAKERY

None

DAIRY

None

CANNED/JARRED GOODS

☐ Pumpkin puree,
  1 (15-ounce) can

☐ Raisins (organic),
  1 (16-ounce) package

☐ Tomato sauce,
  1 (15-ounce) can

☐ Peanut butter (organic),
  1 (16-ounce) jar

☐ Toasted sesame oil,
  1 (8-ounce) bottle

☐ Tamari, 1 (12-ounce) bottle

☐ Hot pepper sesame oil,
  1 (8-ounce) bottle

☐ Brown rice vinegar,
  1 (16-ounce) bottle

☐ Red wine vinegar,
  1 (12-ounce) bottle

☐ Dijon mustard,
  1 (4-ounce) jar

☐ Olive oil (organic),
  1 (16-ounce) bottle

☐ Avocado oil,
  1 (16-ounce) bottle

☐ Black beans, 1 (15-ounce) can

☐ Corn kernels (organic),
1 (15-ounce) can

☐ Balsamic vinegar,
1 (16-ounce) bottle

☐ Chicken broth (organic),
1 (32-ounce) package

☐ Honey (organic),
1 (8-ounce) jar

☐ Japanese rice vinegar
(unseasoned),
1 (8-ounce) bottle

☐ White miso paste
(naturally fermented),
1 (5-ounce) jar

DRIED GOODS/PANTRY ITEMS

☐ Sweetener, like stevia, lo han,
xylitol powder, 1 (1-ounce or
larger) container

☐ Pea protein powder or other
protein base, 14 servings

☐ Chia seeds,
1 (8-ounce) package

☐ Steel-cut or old-fashioned
rolled oats (gluten-free),
1 (32-ounce) package

☐ Almonds,
1 (16-ounce) package

☐ Ceylon cinnamon,
1 (0.5 ounce or larger)
container

☐ Toasted carob powder,
1 (8-ounce) package

☐ Pecan halves (or pieces),
1 (8-ounce) package

☐ Walnut halves (or pieces),
1 (8-ounce) package

☐ Hemp seeds,
1 (8-ounce) package

☐ Fresh or dried turmeric, 1 (0.5-
ounce or larger) container

☐ Natural vanilla extract, 1 (4-
ounce or larger) container

☐ Pumpkin pie spice,
1 (0.5-ounce or larger)
container

☐ Smoked paprika,
1 (0.5-ounce or larger)
container

☐ Pepper, 1 (0.5 ounce or larger)
container

☐ Quinoa, 1 (16-ounce) package

☐ Macadamia nut oil

☐ Cumin seeds, 1 (0.5-ounce or
larger) container

☐ Taco seasoning,
1 (1-ounce) package

☐ Red pepper flakes,
1 (0.5-ounce or larger)
container

☐ Sea salt, 1 (16-ounce) package

☐ Ground cinnamon,
1 (0.5-ounce or larger)
container

☐ Chili powder, 1 (0.5-ounce or
larger) container

☐ White pepper, 1 (0.5-ounce or
larger) container

☐ White sesame seeds,
1 (8-ounce) package

WEEK 2 MENUS	PAGE
DAY 1	
SHAKE Rosemary Pomegranate Blend	128
DINNER Savory and Sweet Stuffed Cabbage	168
UNLIMITED FOOD SUGGESTION Asian Broth	206
DAY 2	
SHAKE Apple Cinnamon Oatmeal	129
DINNER Wild Salmon with Ginger-Lime Marinade	190
UNLIMITED FOOD SUGGESTIONS snow peas and cauliflower florets	
DAY 3	
SHAKE Carob, Pecan, and Banana	130
DINNER Chinese Quinoa Chicken Salad	196
UNLIMITED FOOD SUGGESTION Beet and Fennel Soup	203
DAY 4	
SHAKE Super Red Blend	131
DINNER Seared Cod with Chilled Potatoes	191
UNLIMITED FOOD SUGGESTION celery sticks	
DAY 5	
SHAKE Banana Pumpkin Pie	132
DINNER Potato and Salmon Salad	194
UNLIMITED FOOD SUGGESTION Green Beans with Miso-Sesame Sauce	208
DAY 6	
SHAKE Green Pina Colada	133
DINNER Quinoa Lettuce Wraps	156
UNLIMITED FOOD SUGGESTIONS cherry tomatoes and green onions dipped in sea salt	
DAY 7	
SHAKE Carob Mint	134
DINNER Zucchini Noodles with Baked Shrimp and Tomatoes	186
UNLIMITED FOOD SUGGESTION Zucchini Noodles with Bruschetta	207

WEEK 3 SHOPPING LIST

PRODUCE

- ☐ Banana, 1 medium
- ☐ Lemons, 3
- ☐ Limes, 3
- ☐ Plums, 3 medium
- ☐ Fresh parsley, 1 bunch
- ☐ Oranges, 3
- ☐ Kiwi, 1
- ☐ Fresh cilantro, 2 bunches
- ☐ Fresh ginger, 1 (3-inch) piece
- ☐ Peach, 1 medium
- ☐ Blackberries, 2 pints
- ☐ Garlic, 1 head
- ☐ Green beans (organic), 1½ pounds
- ☐ Grape tomatoes (organic), 2 pints
- ☐ Red onions, 2 medium
- ☐ Cucumber, 1 medium
- ☐ Fresh dill, 1 bunch
- ☐ Fresh mint, 1 bunch

- ☐ Yellow onion, 1 large
- ☐ Arugula, washed leaves, 1 (8-ounce) bag
- ☐ Blueberries or raspberries, 1 pint
- ☐ Beets, 8 medium
- ☐ All-purpose potatoes, 3 medium
- ☐ Carrots, 5 large, 2 medium
- ☐ Broccoli, 1 bunch
- ☐ Shiitake mushrooms, 1 (16-ounce) package
- ☐ Jalapeño, 1
- ☐ Avocado, 1
- ☐ Broccolini, 2 bunches (about 3 pounds)
- ☐ Baby carrots, 1 (16-ounce) package
- ☐ Broccoli florets, 2 (16-ounce) packages
- ☐ Mustard greens, 1 bunch (about 20 ounces)
- ☐ Rosemary, 4 to 6 sprigs

MEAT/FISH

- ☐ Whole chicken, 1 (2–3 pounds)
- ☐ Flank steak (grass-fed), 2½ pounds

- ☐ Chicken breasts, 4 split breasts (about 2 pounds)
- ☐ Chicken sausage (organic), 8 ounces

BEVERAGES

None

FROZEN FOODS

☐ Petite green peas,
1 (16-ounce) package

☐ Blueberries,
1 (16-ounce) package

DAIRY

None

BREAD/BAKERY

None

CANNED/JARRED GOODS

☐ Rosewater,
1 (4-ounce) container

☐ Navy beans, 1 (15-ounce) can

☐ Macadamia nut oil,
1 (16-ounce) bottle

☐ Apple cider vinegar,
1 (16-ounce) bottle

☐ Thai or Vietnamese fish sauce,
1 (8-ounce) bottle

☐ Pumpkin puree
2 (15-ounce) cans

☐ Dill pickles, 1 (16-ounce) jar

☐ Red wine vinegar,
1 (16-ounce) bottle

☐ Whole-grain mustard,
1 (4-ounce) jar

☐ Sardines, 1 (3-ounce) can

☐ Tamari (wheat-free),
1 (12-ounce) bottle

☐ Toasted sesame oil,
1 (8-ounce) bottle

☐ Extra-virgin olive oil,
1 (16-ounce) bottle

☐ Corn kernels,
1 (15-ounce) can

☐ Chicken broth,
1 (32-ounce) container

☐ Avocado oil,
1 (16-ounce) bottle

☐ Unseasoned Japanese rice
vinegar, 1 (8-ounce) bottle

☐ White miso paste
(naturally fermented),
1 (5-ounce) container

DRIED GOODS/PANTRY ITEMS

☐ Sweetener, like stevia, lo han,
xylitol powder,
1 (1-ounce) package

☐ Pea protein powder or other
protein base, 14 servings

☐ Macadamia nuts,
1 (16-ounce) package

☐ Green tea (decaffeinated),
1 package

☐ Chia seeds,
1 (8-ounce) package

☐ Sunflower seeds,
1 (16-ounce) package

☐ Sesame seeds,
1 (8-ounce) package

☐ Almond extract,
1 (1-ounce) bottle

☐ Walnut meats,
1 (16-ounce) bag

☐ Coarse sea salt (iodine-free),
1 (16-ounce) package

☐ Pepper, 1 (0.5-ounce or
larger) container

☐ Arrowroot flour,
1 (0.5-ounce or larger)
container

☐ Ground cumin,
1 (0.5-ounce or larger)
container

☐ Forbidden rice,
1 (16-ounce) package

☐ Cayenne pepper,
1 (0.5-ounce or larger)
container

☐ White sesame seeds,
1 (16-ounce) package

☐ Green banana flour,
1 (16-ounce) package

	WEEK 3 MENUS	PAGE
DAY 1	**SHAKE** Macadamia Green Tea	135
	DINNER Tomato, Cucumber, and Green Bean Salad with Walnut Dressing	192
	UNLIMITED FOOD SUGGESTION Carrot Fries	197
DAY 2	**SHAKE** Blueberry Cheesecake	136
	DINNER Easy Slow Cooker Chicken	184
	UNLIMITED FOOD SUGGESTIONS baby carrots and broccoli florets	
DAY 3	**SHAKE** Green Plum Cooler	137
	DINNER Pumpkin Salad	160
	UNLIMITED FOOD SUGGESTION Sautéed Greens with Lemon	209
DAY 4	**SHAKE** Orange Kiwi Cilantro	138
	DINNER Cold Potato, Beet, Carrot, and Pea Salad with Dill	162
	UNLIMITED FOOD SUGGESTION Beet "Chips"	198
DAY 5	**SHAKE** Peach and Rosewater	139
	DINNER Sesame Beef and Broccoli	182
	UNLIMITED FOOD SUGGESTION broccoli florets	
DAY 6	**SHAKE** Plum Lime Cooler	140
	DINNER Grilled Chicken with Blackberry Salsa	178
	UNLIMITED FOOD SUGGESTION Green Beans with Miso-Sesame Sauce	208
DAY 7	**SHAKE** Blackberry Almond Chia	141
	DINNER Broccolini Chicken and Rice	173
	UNLIMITED FOOD SUGGESTION Beet "Chips"	198

WEEK 4 SHOPPING LIST

PRODUCE

- [ ] Limes, 4
- [ ] Blood orange, 1
- [ ] Fresh ginger, 1 (3-inch) piece
- [ ] Bananas, 3 medium
- [ ] Dark cherries, 1 (16-ounce) package
- [ ] Fresh spinach, 2 (6-ounce) bags
- [ ] Swiss chard, 1 bunch
- [ ] Avocado, 1
- [ ] Fresh cilantro, 2 bunches
- [ ] Fresh parsley, 2 bunches
- [ ] Raspberries, 1 pint
- [ ] Peach, 1 medium
- [ ] Garlic, 4 heads
- [ ] Green beans (organic), $1/2$ pound
- [ ] Grape tomatoes (organic), 1 pint
- [ ] Red onion, 1 medium
- [ ] Cucumbers, 3 large
- [ ] Fresh dill, 1 bunch
- [ ] Fresh mint, 1 bunch
- [ ] Fresh thyme, 2 bunches
- [ ] Cherry tomatoes, 2 pints
- [ ] Carrots, 6 large
- [ ] Celery, 1 bunch

- [ ] Yellow onions, 4 large
- [ ] Zucchinis, 2 medium
- [ ] Fresh basil, 1 bunch
- [ ] Lettuce (butter or iceberg), 2 heads
- [ ] Tomatoes, 4 medium
- [ ] Bok choy, 1 bunch with 4 to 6 stems and leaves
- [ ] Mushrooms, 2 (16-ounce) packages
- [ ] Green onions, 1 bunch
- [ ] Snow peas, 1 (16-ounce) package
- [ ] Baby carrots, 1 (16-ounce) package
- [ ] Red bell pepper, 1
- [ ] Onions, 2 medium
- [ ] Fresh tarragon, 1 bunch
- [ ] Lemons, 2
- [ ] Shiitake mushrooms, 2 (16-ounce) packages
- [ ] Lemongrass, 1 stalk
- [ ] Beets, 4 medium
- [ ] Fennel bulb, 1
- [ ] Cauliflower florets, 1 package

MEAT/FISH

☐ Skinless, boneless chicken breasts (organic), 1½ pounds

☐ White fish fillets of choice, 1 pound

☐ Lean ground turkey (organic), 1 pound

BEVERAGES

☐ Cooking wine of choice, 1 bottle

☐ Tomato juice, 2 (16-ounce) cans

DAIRY

None

FROZEN FOODS

☐ Blueberries, 1 (16-ounce) package

BREAD/BAKERY

Rice tortillas, 1 (10-ounce) package

CANNED/JARRED GOODS

☐ Macadamia nut oil, 1 (16-ounce) bottle

☐ White kidney beans, 1 (15-ounce) can

☐ Apple cider vinegar, 1 (8-ounce) bottle

☐ Chickpeas, 1 (15-ounce) can

☐ Thai or Vietnamese fish sauce, 1 (8-ounce) bottle

☐ Diced tomatoes, 1 (15-ounce) can

☐ Olive oil, 1 (16-ounce) bottle

☐ Chicken broth (organic), 2 (32-ounce) containers

☐ Red kidney beans, 1 (15-ounce) can

☐ Coconut milk, 1 (15-ounce) can

☐ Avocado oil,
   1 (8-ounce) bottle

☐ Pinto beans,
   1 (15-ounce) can

☐ Soy sauce,
   1 (12-ounce) bottle

☐ Teriyaki sauce
   (gluten-free),
   1 (8-ounce) jar

☐ Sweet chili sauce,
   1 (8-ounce) bottle

☐ Vegetable broth,
   1 (32-ounce) container

☐ Pumpkin puree,
   1 (15-ounce) can

☐ Red wine vinegar,
   1 (16-ounce) bottle

☐ Tomato paste,
   1 (6-ounce) can

☐ Honey (organic),
   1 (8-ounce) jar

DRIED GOODS/PANTRY ITEMS

☐ Sweetener, like stevia,
   lo han, xylitol powder,
   1 (1-ounce) package

☐ Pea protein powder, or other
   protein base, 14 servings

☐ Chia seeds,
   1 (8-ounce) package

☐ Coarse sea salt,
   1 (16-ounce) package

☐ Pepper, 1 (0.5-ounce or larger)
   container

☐ Sunflower seeds,
   1 (16-ounce) package

☐ Carob powder,
   1 (4-ounce) package

☐ Tiger nuts,
   1 (8-ounce) package

☐ Green banana flour,
   1 (16-ounce) package

☐ Brazil nuts,
   1 (8-ounce) package

☐ Peppermint essential oil
   (food-grade),
   1 (1-ounce) bottle

☐ Cardamom in the pod,
   1 (1-ounce) jar

☐ Vanilla extract,
   1 (4-ounce jar)

☐ Walnut meats,
   1 (16-ounce) bag

☐ Pasta (gluten-free),
   1 (16-ounce) package

☐ Sunflower seeds,
   1 (16-ounce) package

☐ Nutritional yeast (folic acid-
   free), 1 (16-ounce) package

☐ Arrowroot powder,
   1 (16-ounce) package

☐ Almonds,
   1 (16-ounce) package

☐ Onion powder

☐ Brown rice,
   1 (16-ounce) package

☐ Cashews,
   1 (8-ounce) package

☐ Dry mustard,
   1 (1-ounce) container

☐ Granulated garlic,
   1 (0.5-ounce or larger)
   container

☐ Ground ginger,
   1 (0.5-ounce or larger)
   container

☐ Arborio rice,
   1 (16-ounce) package

☐ Ground nutmeg,
   1 (0.5-ounce or larger)
   container

☐ Cayenne pepper,
   1 (0.5-ounce or larger)
   container

☐ Red pepper flakes,
   1 (0.5-ounce or larger)
   container

☐ Ground cinnamon,
   1 (0.5-ounce or larger)
   container

☐ Chili powder,
   1 (0.5-ounce or larger)
   container

☐ White pepper,
   1 (0.5-ounce or larger)
   container

☐ Ground cumin,
   1 (0.5-ounce or larger)
   container

WEEK 4 MENUS	PAGE
SHAKE Blueberry Lime Smoothie	142
DINNER Tomato, Cucumber, and Green Bean Salad with Walnut Dressing	192
UNLIMITED FOOD SUGGESTION snow peas	
SHAKE Blood Orange Sunflower Smoothie	143
DINNER Unbeatable Minestrone	176
UNLIMITED FOOD SUGGESTION baby carrots	
SHAKE Black Forest Cherry Smoothie	144
DINNER Creamy Basil and Chicken	174
UNLIMITED FOOD SUGGESTION Fresh Spring Gazpacho	202
SHAKE Green Power Smoothie	145
DINNER Sprouted-Almond Fish "Taco" Bowl	154
UNLIMITED FOOD SUGGESTION Asian Broth	206
SHAKE Raspberry Tigernut Blast	146
DINNER Asian Chicken Bowl	153
UNLIMITED FOOD SUGGESTION Beet and Fennel Soup	203
SHAKE Peppermint Brazil Nut Smoothie	147
DINNER Healthy Turkey Lettuce Wraps	158
UNLIMITED FOOD SUGGESTIONS cucumber slices and cauliflower florets	
SHAKE Cardamom Peach	150
DINNER Vegan Pumpkin Risotto	170
UNLIMITED FOOD SUGGESTION Chili-Roasted Carrots	199

Day rows (left column): DAY 1, DAY 2, DAY 3, DAY 4, DAY 5, DAY 6, DAY 7

Now you know exactly what to eat for your Reset! But don't forget that these recipes and guidelines are only part of the Reset. The diet works best when you match it with a healthy lifestyle. Please join me for the next chapter, and you will learn about how to sleep and lounge your way to metabolism repair.

chapter six

Reset Lifestyle

Diet is the foundation of the Reset, and with a few simple tips, you can amplify the results and make sure your healthy new metabolism will last. This means you will drop more inches, have fewer cravings, and step off the diet roller-coaster for good.

Of the lifestyle tips, the most powerful may be as simple as to get a good night's sleep.

SLEEP

In traditional Chinese medicine, lack of sleep was considered one of the main causes of liver disease. Today we know this idea has merit. During the daytime, your liver is working hard to manage the food you eat and convert it to energy to power your mental and physical activities. Only during deep sleep does your liver get the break it needs to refill its glycogen supplies. When it cannot refill glycogen, you lose your metabolic flexibility because your liver can no longer burn its stored triglycerides.

Sleep issues come in three main forms: (1) people do not make sleep a priority, (2) they cannot get to sleep, or (3) they cannot stay asleep. To make sleep a priority, it may help to realize that many experts think sleep affects your figure more than either exercise or diet.[1] Since the 1980s, we have experienced an epidemic of inadequate sleep. More people than ever work with teams in different time zones or answer emails outside the normal workday. Restful sleep is an essential step toward a successful reset of your liver and moving into a naturally lean life.

Missing a single night's sleep can make a normal person crave more food, prefer worse quality food, and loathe the idea of exercise. There are also valid vanity reasons—science has shown that sleep can contribute to collagen synthesis more than creams, lotions, or potions. Beauty sleep is a real thing![2]

If you have had a hard time falling asleep, you will likely do better during the Reset program, for many reasons. The combo of RS and protein keeps your blood sugar from dropping at night, and the break from caffeine and alcohol can make a big difference. The journaling helps also. The sleep rituals that follow can help further if sleep is still an issue.

When people are able to initially fall asleep just fine, but they wake up too early, the culprit is usually a drop in blood sugar. Your body uses cortisol to raise your blood sugar when it drops off at night. Normally, cortisol is low while you are sleeping, and you make a bunch to wake yourself up in the morning. If you make too much cortisol before it is time to wake up, you may suddenly feel wide awake with your mind racing about some possible calamity. In the moment, it feels like whatever situation your mind settled on was the cause. There is always something the mind can stew over; we could have said that one thing differently, or we should not have missed out on that other thing. But it was really your blood sugar and cortisol that made it happen.

The Reset foods are rich in RS, which keeps your blood sugar from these sudden drop-offs. If you still wake early or often, an easy trick is a half serving of an RS food right at bedtime. Try half a boiled potato or half a serving of the original Reset Shake (one scoop instead of two; see page 119). The RS is not a sedative, but it keeps your blood sugar from dropping for seven to nine hours and lets you sleep soundly through the night.

SLEEP RITUALS

All parents who have had small children know that if the child's night-time routine becomes disrupted, the whole house is in for a poor night's sleep. As adults, we often fail to realize that we are just as dependent on rituals to give us deep and refreshing sleep.

UPON WAKING

How you sleep is largely affected by how you wake. What you do in the first hour of your morning can make or break the quality of your sleep the following night. The most important step of all is this: make sure to wake up at the same time every day.

Here is how it can go wrong. You have to wake up for work, for your kid's school, or for your school earlier than you would like, but on the weekend, you sleep in. What happens is that your body thinks that morning should arrive no sooner than the latest you woke up in the last four to five days.

As an example, say that on Saturday and Sunday you wake up at 9 a.m. On Monday, Tuesday, and Wednesday, when you wake up at 6 a.m., it is just like you have jet lag. In fact, the condition is called "social jet lag." Those who have it usually start their week feeling sluggish, partially checked out, and just counting hours until the weekend. By Friday, they may start to feel better. Now comes the weekend, and the cycle starts all over again.

The solution may not be easy, but it is simple and I promise sleep is worth it. Figure out how late you can sleep during the week and still do all your morning routines like exercise, breakfast, grooming, and commuting. Try to find some parts of this you can do in advance. Even a few easy steps to getting breakfast ready or laying out your clothes will make your morning more efficient and less stressful. Once you know how late you can sleep, make that your wake-up time throughout the week. During your reset, your mornings will be especially smooth because preparing your first few meals is incredibly simple and exercise takes only a few minutes.

Of course, it will be tempting to get extra sleep the first few weekends—*do not do it*. If you feel tired later in the day, feel free to take a nap, but still wake up at your set time in the morning. You will start to go to bed earlier, spontaneously. You will also feel more rested and find that you are losing weight and feeling more energetic.

Along with waking up at the same time, the two other morning rituals that will help are eating an early breakfast and getting some bright light first thing in the morning.

EARLY BREAKFAST

Be sure to have your breakfast shake within an hour of waking up. If you have been in the habit of missing breakfast or having it later in the morning, you may be surprised by how much this one small change can improve your day and give you steadier energy levels and fewer cravings.

BRIGHT LIGHT

Have you ever noticed how when you are camping you naturally wake up with the sun? There is a hormonal event called the *cortisol awakening response* that is triggered by sunlight and wakes you up in the morning. Even though we have plenty of lights inside our homes, artificial lights and even sunny rooms lack the intensity and the wavelengths of direct natural sunlight.

Light intensity is measured in a unit called a lux. One lux is the light intensity of a typical candle from 1 meter (roughly 3 feet) in a dark room.[3] Most homes and office buildings range from 50 to 80 lux of light intensity, whereas outdoors on a cloudy day may be over 1,000 lux. The light intensity outside in the shade may be 25,000 lux and direct sun can be as high as 130,000. It seems that our brains require roughly 10,000 lux to register that it is time to trigger the cortisol awakening response and start the day.

How can you get 10,000 lux? Just spend as little as 30 minutes outdoors soon after waking. To be precise, you do not need to be in direct sunlight, nor do you need your skin exposed. Bronzing in the Speedo is not mandatory. Your eyes just need the light, so they can send a signal to your pineal gland, which connects to your adrenals. Your adrenals respond to this light and make a healthy burst of cortisol so that you feel awake.

You can be in a shaded area but you will get the best effects if you do not wear sunglasses. When the weather allows, do as much of your morning ritual as you can outdoors—have your shake, take a walk, or just read and relax.

Based on your latitude and the time of year, sometimes it is still dark for some time after you wake up. If this is true for you, consider having your breakfast while basking in the light of a light therapy box. Look for units that emit 10,000 lux and do not create UV or blue light.

Light therapies are most effective when the source of light is higher than your eyes. One can sit in a chair next to a floor lamp or work at a table with a table lamp that is several feet above the table's surface. Please note that there are some medical conditions like bipolar disorder or diabetic retinopathy with which light therapy can be counterproductive. Check with your health provider to be sure that light therapy is safe for you.

EVENING RITUALS

Here are some steps to take at nighttime to give you better sleep:

90 minutes before bed

- Lower the temperature in your home by 5 degrees Fahrenheit or roughly 3 degrees Celsius.
- Make a hot cup of chamomile or lemon balm tea.

60 minutes before bed

- Turn off computers, TV screens, and LED display screens.
- Turn off any extra lights.
- Take a quick shower with warm but not hot water.
- Turn on a source of white noise like a white noise generator, an app, a fan, or a HEPA air filter.

10 minutes before bed

- Write in your journal.

HOW TO JOURNAL

The journaling helps because your brain stores trauma, unfinished actions, and powerful memories in areas that can trigger strong emotions and subconscious stress responses. Often these unresolved events can trigger anxiety for no apparent reason. When you convert your feelings into words, it prompts a neurologic change. MRI scans have proven that the act of speaking or writing about feelings that are top of mind can move stored experiences away from the emotional reptilian parts of the brain, where they continually recirculate up to the rational parts of the brain, where they begin to dissipate. This effect can be invoked any time you convert ideas into words, regardless of whether you are speaking, writing, or typing and regardless of any feedback you receive.

How do you begin to journal? Use your Reset journal or a computer app. Many mobile apps for journaling are available but many people have an easier time with writing or typing on a keyboard. My personal favorite journaling app is called *Day One*. Whatever method you use, make sure it will remain private for your use only. Even if you have no fearsome secrets, you will be able to write more freely if you do not need to wonder how your writings would sound to someone else.

Start a timer set for 5 minutes and simply write whatever comes to mind. Do not worry about grammar, syntax, spelling, or construction. Feel free to follow from one thought to the next. The act of writing them is qualitatively more cathartic than simply letting them ruminate in your mind.

Sometimes you may write about trivialities of recent memory. Some sessions may include memories of trauma. Some may be about aspirations. Do not judge the content, just keep writing. If you wish to finish a thought or idea after the timer has gone off, feel free to do so.

Sweet dreams!

EXERCISE

Of those who attempted the Reset but did not get the full benefits the first time through, nearly all were over-exercising. I know we have all been led to believe that we need to train hard to lose adipose tissue, but I have seen this promise fall flat for myself and so many others that it is time to put it to rest.

Please do hear the full message: exercise is good. In fact, it has no equal in terms of its benefits for brain performance, disease prevention, and a healthy mood. It is one of my favorite things in life and the evidence supporting it is monumental.

You will exercise during the Reset, but please know that the program will not work as well if you do more than recommended. The Metabolism Reset activates your muscle tissue so that it can work with your liver to become a backup storage location for extra fuel. If you did hard exercise during the Reset, your liver would have to manage so much fuel that it would not get the chance to repair. If you did no exercise, your muscles would become dormant and end up getting used as a source of protein.

Before starting any new exercise regime, check with your health provider to be sure these activities are appropriate for you!

GENTLE MOVEMENT

Each day, expect the majority of your exercise time to be spent walking. Please use a pedometer, fitness tracker, your phone, or your smartwatch to track your steps. Believe it or not, the goal during the Reset will be to not take too many steps. The lower limit is 5,000 steps and the upper limit is 10,000. You may have read of recommendations to do more than 10,000 steps daily. This can be great for everyday life, but is too much for our purposes right now. Our goal is to keep your blood moving but not to burn lots of extra fuel.

Start each day with a brief morning walk of 1,000 to 3,000 steps. Based on your pace and stride length, this will likely take 10 to 20 minutes. Use your step counter for the rest of the day also. Your routine activities will typically give an additional 2,000 to 7,000 steps.

MICRO WORKOUTS

There are two micro workouts on the Reset program—one is intervals, the other is a sequence of bodyweight exercises. Do one workout each day in alternation—intervals on odd-numbered days, and bodyweight exercises on even-numbered days, for example. These are considered micro workouts because you will be able to complete them in under 5 minutes.

INTERVALS

You can do intervals by jogging or cycling outdoors or indoors on a treadmill, exercise bike, elliptical trainer, or stair-stepper. After you have warmed up, go for 20 seconds at full intensity, followed by 40 seconds at an easy pace. You can raise the intensity by going faster, going uphill, or adding resistance to a machine. Complete three cycles of fast and slow finishing with the slow 40 seconds.

If you plan on doing your interval workout on a bike or aerobic machine, you can skip your walk and instead do an easy 10 to 20 minutes as a warmup.

Walking example

1. Do your daily 10- to 20-minute casual walk to warm up.
2. Walk, jog, or run as fast as you comfortably can for 20 seconds.
3. Go as slow as you wish for 40 seconds.
4. Repeat steps 2 and 3 for 3 times total, finishing with step 3.
5. You are all done!

Exercise bike example

1. Ride for 10 to 20 minutes with little or no resistance.
2. Increase the resistance and ride at a challenging pace for 20 seconds.
3. Ride slowly without resistance for 40 seconds.
4. Repeat steps 2 and 3 for 3 times total, finishing with step 3.
5. That is it!

BODYWEIGHT ROUTINE

Equipment needed—not much at all. You can wear any comfortable and loose clothes. You can do this workout with or without shoes because there is no jumping or impact. Just be sure you have a soft carpet or an exercise/yoga mat. You will need enough space to lie down and stretch out. It helps to have a visible clock that has a second hand.

You will do a total of five exercises. Do each one for 30 seconds and then rest for 30 seconds before moving on to the next. The exercises are in an intended sequence—do them in order, starting with no. 1 and finishing with no. 5.

Since you are timing each step, the routine will take exactly 5 minutes to complete. In case you are getting back into shape or really fit already, there are variations after the description of each exercise so that you can make it more comfortable or more challenging.

If you are super-fit, feel free to do all the hard variations—just keep it to 5 minutes total.

EXERCISES

1. Air squats

STARTING POSITION Stand with your feet shoulder-width apart. Extend your arms in front of you and lower your seat until your thighs are parallel with the floor. Completed Position: Return to starting position. Repeat as many as you can for 30 seconds.

If it is too hard at first:
- Hold on to a wall for balance.
- Do not go down all the way.
- Do the exercise over a chair so you will not go down too far.
- Stop before the full 30 seconds.

If it is way too easy:
- Go faster.
- Squat more deeply, try to touch your rear-end to the ground.

- Move for 45 seconds instead of 30.
- Hold a weighted dumbbell in each hand.

2. Push-ups

STARTING POSITION Lie on a carpet or exercise mat facedown with your body straight and your hands on the floor under your armpits with your elbows bent. Straighten your arms raising your body straight off of the ground, supporting your weight on your knees or your feet. Completed Position: Return to starting position. Repeat as many as you can for 30 seconds.

If it is too hard at first:
- Rather than lying on the floor, lean against a stable desk or table with your feet on the floor.
- Do not go down all the way.
- Stop before the full 30 seconds.

If it is way too easy:
- Go faster.
- Move for 45 seconds instead of 30.
- Elevate your feet on a stable surface while keeping your hands on the floor.

3. Stationary lunges

STARTING POSITION Stand up straight with your feet shoulder-width apart and your hands laced behind your neck. Step forward and bend your rear leg, tapping the knee on your rear leg gently on the floor. Completed Position: Return to starting position and repeat with opposite leg forward. Repeat as many as you can for 30 seconds.

If it is too hard at first:
- Hold on to a wall for balance.
- Do not go down all the way.
- Stop before the full 30 seconds.

If it is way too easy:

- Go faster.
- Move for 45 seconds instead of 30.
- Hold a weighted dumbbell in each hand.

4. Reverse snow angels

If you did not grow up with snow, you might not know what a snow angel is. I sure made my share in northern Minnesota. In a normal snow angel, you lie flat on your back in the snow and open and close your arms and legs. If you do it right, you end up with an impression that vaguely looks like an angel's gown, wings, and head. We will do the same on our stomachs instead; snow is entirely optional.

STARTING POSITION Lie on your abdomen with your legs straight and your arms together straight at your sides. Lift your arms and legs off the ground. Move your arms from your side to overhead while you extend your legs as far as you can away from your centerline. Completed Position: Return to starting position. Repeat as many as you can for 30 seconds.

If it is too hard at first:

- Just move your arms—only move them as far as you can.
- Stop before the full 30 seconds.

If it is way too easy:

- Go faster.
- Move for 45 seconds instead of 30.

5. Plank

STARTING POSITION Lie on a carpet or exercise mat facedown with your body straight and your hands on the floor under your armpits with your elbows bent. Straighten your arms, raising your body straight off of the ground, supporting your weight on your hands and knees (easier) or your feet (more advanced). Completed Position: Hold this position with your body straight for 30 seconds.

If it is too hard at first:
- Elevate your hands with a stable platform like a table or counter.
- Stop before the full 30 seconds.

If it is way too easy:
- Elevate your feet with a stable platform like a table or counter.
- Move for 45 seconds instead of 30.

For each week during your four-week Reset, alternate your daily exercise from bodyweight to intervals, always including your walk.

SUPPLEMENTS

If you are like most health-consumers, you have a cupboard full of supplements. There are a few you take every day, some you take if you notice the bottle, and some you take if you think of a specific concern. Whatever you put in your mouth ultimately goes to your liver first. Certain medications or supplements are known to be harmful to the liver, but some combinations can also harm it in ways that you would not expect.

I have seen many cases of patients who had liver damage due to taking large numbers of supplements. They had a list that grew from their own interests or from the recommendations of another practitioner. This harm can happen even when none of the individual nutrients are ones that are known to be toxic to the liver. Remember that the liver is a filter and a buffer. When a large number of highly concentrated chemicals enters in amounts much beyond what would be found in food, it can place your liver under strain.

Sometimes the number of pills a person takes creeps up inadvertently. You may have started taking a pill on your own or been prescribed one for reasons that are no longer relevant. Perhaps you see multiple health-care providers. In many cases, a doctor may prescribe a pill without knowing or thinking about the other pills you are already taking. Unfortunately, many people are given pills to counteract side effects from another pill that they do not even need to take.

On your next visit with your primary-care provider, bring all your pills with you and talk to her or him about each one. Sometimes doctors gloss over a list of pills on paper but take notice when they actually see them all together. If you take prescription medicines on a daily basis, please ask your doctor if you really need to and if so, how you could make them unnecessary. And please do not stop taking any medications or supplements that a doctor prescribed for you without speaking to her or him about it.

With that in mind, there are some essential nutrients that are hard to get, even from the healthiest diet. There are also accessory nutrients and plant extracts that can help your liver break down the trapped triglycerides that are holding back your metabolism.

MULTIVITAMINS

During the four-week Reset, your food intake will be reduced and your body could run low on essential micronutrients at a time when your body may need them more than ever. Choose a 30-day supply of a good multivitamin/multimineral with the following considerations:

IRON-FREE

Iron makes other minerals in the same pill hard to absorb. Important nutrients like zinc, selenium, and magnesium do not absorb as well when they are included in a pill that has iron. Besides the absorption problems, iron can be dangerous for those who do not need it. If your doctor says that you need iron, take it in a separate pill from your multivitamins. Iron supplements can cause constipation and digestive distress because they are hard to absorb. A form of iron called iron bisglycinate may be absorbed best and least apt to cause digestive side effects.

WITHOUT FOLIC ACID

Folic acid is a synthetic form of a group of naturally occurring B-vitamins called folates. Many people are genetically unable to process synthetic folic acid. Not only can they not make use of it, but it can block the good effects of natural folates. Synthetic folic acid can also impair liver function and raise the risk of colorectal cancer.[4] Better multivitamins use only natural versions of folate such as methyl folate.

IODINE-FREE

Iodine is an essential mineral. If you get less than 50 mcg daily, your thyroid cannot work as well. Thankfully, you would have to do some serious planning to get less than this. The odd thing is that you can also get too much. In fact, the thyroid can also be stressed with above as little as 300 mcg daily. Few if any nutrients have such a narrow range of safety. Those who are on thyroid medications also get a fair amount from their thyroid pill. Typically, they are already at the upper limit of what is safe between their medication and their diet.

Raw-food vegans who use iodine-free salt and no sea vegetables can be at risk of iodine deficiency. Nearly everyone else can easily get 150 to 200 mcg from their diet. For the millions of people who have thyroid disease and the millions more who are prone to it, extra iodine from vitamins is best to avoid. Too much iodine can slow thyroid function, which hurts the basal metabolic rate.

This step is so important that one study showed that 78 percent of people who were hypothyroid due to Hashimoto's could be cured by doing nothing else besides restricting their iodine intake to these guidelines.[5]

SAFE CALCIUM

Most forms of calcium supplements raise the risk for heart attacks more than they lower the risk of osteoporosis.[6] Calcium carbonate, oyster shell calcium, and coral calcium are especially problematic. Only use vitamins that are based on safe forms of protein-chelated calcium, such as calcium dicalcium malate, or calcium glycinate. These forms of calcium are also better absorbed so fewer milligrams are needed. The ideal dose in supplements is 300 to 500 mg.

ADDITIONAL LIVER SUPPORT OPTIONS

If your Metabolism Quiz score (see page 5) was over 4, you may also consider adaptogens for liver support. These are food-like ingredients that are safe and easy to include. Here are a few liver helpers to consider and reasons why they can help.

MUSHROOMS

Reishi

Shown to protect human liver cells against damage from chemical stressors and free radicals.[7]

Cordyceps

An exotic fungi that grows only at high elevations in the cocoons of silkworms. Used for a tonic since as early as 5000 BCE.[8] Known to protect liver and kidney cells and improve their ability to form energy.[9]

BOTANICAL EXTRACTS

Schisandra berry (Schisandra chinensis)

Also known as wu wei zi or "berry of 5 flavors." Extracts of this berry have been shown to prevent the buildup of triglycerides within liver cells and help dissolve triglycerides that are trapped.[10] They have also been shown to reverse the exact type of damage to the liver cell's endoplasmic reticulum that makes the cells unable to break down stored triglycerides for energy.[11]

Burdock root (Arctium lappa)

This plant has been shown to have over 11 constituents that protect the liver and help it remove trapped triglycerides and cholesterol.[12] It is also called gobo root and has been used as a food in Japanese cuisine for centuries.

Milk thistle seed (Silybum marianum)

Milk thistle seeds have been used for centuries in Europe and America as a treatment for liver and gallbladder disorders. Numerous human studies have shown multiple benefits they may have on liver function including:

- Delays the formation of liver fibrosis
- Acts as an antioxidant
- Lowers levels of liver inflammation
- Reduces triglycerides within the liver
- Improves insulin sensitivity
- Helps the liver burn fuel more efficiently[13,14]

Milk thistle seeds can be taken as a food or in supplement form. When the whole seeds are used, they should be ground or blended since they are usually too hard to chew safely.

You should now have a clear sense of the importance of sleep, stress reduction, exercise, and taking the right pills. Please dial in these lifestyle habits for your Reset so that you can make the benefits of a healthy metabolism last for you.

BONUS: MENTAL RESET

If you have a high level of stress in your life, here is an optional way you can help prevent it from sabotaging your Reset.

It is no secret that stress is hard on you in every way. More evidence supports that it also hurts the metabolism. Your stress hormones act on your liver to keep it in a storage mode and make it unable to burn tri-glycerides. In fact, under chronic stress, your liver actually amplifies your stress hormones, making them even more harmful. Sadly, many assume that, as harmful as stress is, there is little we can do about it. In order to reduce stress, it often feels as if one would need to change their lives in ways that are not realistic or spend inordinate amounts of time on difficult mind–body techniques that only lead to frustration.

Thankfully, you can get measurable benefits with a simple technique that takes only 5 minutes.

VISUAL FOCUS

Are you not a natural meditator? Many find it hard to close their eyes and focus on their breath or a word. If you have ever struggled with a racing mind while you tried to quiet it, this may be a great exercise for you. You do not need to try to control your mind at all. All you do is focus your vision. Try it for 5 minutes before breakfast.

Select a quiet location in which you can sit comfortably and you will not be disturbed. Sit with your spine straight. You can use a chair but try not to lean against its back. You can also kneel on the floor or sit in a lotus or half-lotus posture.

Place an object on which to focus your visual attention on the floor 4 to 6 feet in front of you. Traditional Yogis used a lit candle, but LED candles also work. You can even use one of many apps that show a simulated candle flame. Get a timer set for 5 minutes. The basic technique is to focus a soft gaze on the tip of the candle while keeping your back straight. Once you are settled in, activate the 5-minute timer. Breathe deeply into your abdomen through your nose if possible.

Do not worry about your mind racing or wandering around. It is normal to have frequent thoughts and sensations from your body. You may find yourself looking away or letting your attention drift to objects in the periphery of your vision. This is also normal. Once you notice you have done so, simply return your gaze to the candle.

Ancient Yogis called this technique Trataka, which means "to look."

The act of visual focus helps you identify space between your awareness and your thought. You start to realize that your thoughts are not generated from "you" but, rather, are events that come and go in your mind on their own accord.

The benefits spill over into life outside of the practice. The next time you get wrapped up in distressful thoughts, you may automatically just focus on a point in your visual field and take a few breaths. You can deal with any immediate concern more effectively when you are able to let your thoughts come and go without taking them seriously.

A DAY IN THE RESET

Let's put the whole thing together and see how a day looks. To make it clear how these various parts of the program work in harmony, the following is an overview of a typical day during the Reset.

TIME TO START YOUR DAY!

As you wake up you can start the day feeling good about yourself because you are doing what your body needs so that you can feel healthier. During your Reset, get in the habit of waking up at the same time every day rather than sleeping in on the weekends. This habit may be one of the most important toward achieving your goals.

HYDRATION

Start your day with an 8-ounce glass of purified water with a splash of lemon juice. Hydration is critical for elimination of wastes. Your liver will be processing lots of trapped triglycerides and adipose tissue in the coming days. Imagine your liver working like a garbage disposal. If there is no water flowing through it, everything gets gummed up.

RESTROOM

Your first order of business will be to use the restroom. Most people will have their main bowel movement soon after waking up and at least once daily. If yours are less frequent than daily, or if it takes so long that you have made your restroom into an office, please visit Chapter 10 ("FAQ").

BREAKFAST

Have your first shake within an hour of waking up. Use the Shake Assembly Guide in Chapter 5 or choose a shake recipe in Chapter 7. Do you have a full schedule for the day? If so, you may as well make it a double. Mix up the second batch of your shake at the same time if your blender has room, or right after making the first. Now you don't have to worry about your lunch prep.

Along with your shake, pour your second glass of water to work on throughout the morning or bring with you while you are out.

Note: Are you in the first few days of your Reset? Do you know you are going to get hungry? If so, make sure you have some anytime snacks prepped and packed for the day. Learn more about them in Chapter 8.

EXERCISE

Get your blood flowing with a short, gentle walk lasting 10 to 20 minutes. If you can, walk to work! On odd calendar days, follow your walk with the interval micro workout (page 104) and on even days with the bodyweight routine. Visit metabolismresetdietbook.com for exercise videos. Be sure to drink another glass of water when you finish.

MID-MORNING

Have another 8-ounce glass of water. If you feel hungry, have some unlimited foods as needed.

LUNCH

Start with another 8-ounce glass of water while you get your shake together, then enjoy your shake.

You might be surprised at how easy it is to get into the groove of a couple of favorite recipes, or even one. That is fine. It is nice to have a break from thinking so much about food. Of course, you always have the option of trying out new recipes and exotic ingredients if you choose to.

MID-AFTERNOON

The same drill as mid-morning—have some more water and unlimited foods as needed. Most people notice that their afternoon hunger drops off even sooner than their mid-morning hunger. If your hunger ever seems unbearable, be sure to visit Chapter 10 ("FAQ").

DINNER

Okay, now it is time for the main meal. Even if it seems like a lot of food, please finish it and enjoy it. Have your last glass of water for the day with your dinner.

Note: If your days are busy, be sure to keep prepped veggies and batches of cooked good carbs and proteins ready in advance for the week.

UNWINDING

By now, your day's activity has wound down. After you have cleaned up the kitchen, you probably want to unwind for a bit. It is no coincidence that words like "stress," "tension," "relax," and "unwind" can relate to your feelings, as well as your muscles. Some are in the habit of using alcohol to lower the tension that built up throughout the day. Yes, wine is still alcohol, even if you only drink it because you like the taste.

After dinner, take a quick walk. Even 10 minutes at a casual pace will go a long way toward lowering the day's stress hormones. You might spend the last act of your day reading, watching television, or surfing the web. Whatever you do, see if it is more relaxing when paired with the effortless stretches described earlier in this chapter. For the first

10 minutes of vegging out, do it while you are stretching, and see if your mind feels more at ease.

BEDTIME

Remember that sleep is the third part of the recovery. Plan on at least eight hours of sleep during the Reset. Since this may involve going to bed earlier than you are used to, treat yourself like a baby and start your evening ritual ninety minutes before bed. See the details of the ritual on page 99. Is it hard to fall asleep or stay asleep through the night? If so, .be sure to check the tips earlier in this chapter.

How can you hold on to the transformation and not slip back to an inflexible metabolism? My experience has taught me that most find it easier than they expect. You are probably already doing many of the habits that will keep your liver from getting clogged up. In the next chapter, I will give you a good overview of how you can live your life without obsessing over food and still keep your metabolism healthy.

chapter seven

Shake Recipes

You can complete your Reset with either premade shakes or ones you assemble in your own kitchen. The advantage of assembling your own shake is that you can choose ingredients from your local supermarket and sample from the many recipes found in this section. The advantage of using a premade product is that you can be assured to receive the exact ingredients used in the Metabolism Reset Diet clinical trials and reduce time spent on shopping and food preparation.

To learn more about the original Reset Shake used in our clinical trials, visit metabolismresetdietbook.com/resources.

HOW TO MAKE YOUR RESET SHAKE

The main goals behind the reset shake are to have 23 or more grams of high-quality protein, 20,000 mg or more of RS, a low-acid-residue pH, and no refined sugar, no artificial colors or flavorings, no folic acid, and under 20 mcg of iodine.

. . .

There are enough recipes in this chapter so you can have a new shake on every day of your Reset. Please know that you have a variety of options available, but you do not need to make every single one.

Most people find a handful of recipes that appeal to them because they have flavors they know they prefer. From these, they often make several of their top favorites and rely upon them throughout the Reset.

Each recipe makes two servings. As mentioned earlier, the best idea is to make the whole recipe and use half as your breakfast shake and half as your lunch shake. You can also make the full batch and share half with a loved one who is doing the Reset with you. You can also use half the recipe and refrigerate the remainder in the blender bowl or a glass container. Just be sure to mix well again and drink within 48 hours. If you wish to make a single serving, simply reduce all of the ingredients by 50 percent.

Should you use organic ingredients? Some ingredients are more important to choose organic than others. For example, consider choosing organic whenever the peel of a plant is used as food or the recipe uses plants known to be particularly high in pesticide residues. I suggest organic in these cases for the recipes. You can never go wrong with choosing organic anytime; but if that is not an option, do not let the perfect be the enemy of the good. You are still better off eating more produce, not less, even if it is not all organic.

To make these smoothies, you'll need a blender and a flexible spatula. Add the ingredients in the order listed. If the mixture isn't blending completely, turn the power off and use the flexible spatula to scrape down the sides of the blender bowl, then turn the power back on and blend until smooth.

Strawberry Orange Sunrise

PREP TIME: 5 MINUTES
MAKES 2 SERVINGS

This works really well with frozen strawberries. Frozen fruit is just as "fresh," or often even fresher, than fresh fruit that may have been sitting around for a while. It is also usually less costly, has a longer shelf life, and requires no preparation. I normally use navel oranges, but the zest from any variety of orange works well.

- 1 cup purified water

- 1 cup ice cubes

- RS supplement (1 serving) or RS food ($1/4$ cup green banana flour, $1/2$ cup aquafaba, or others on page 64)

- Sweetener to taste (stevia or lo han)

- 1 cup (organic) strawberries, washed and trimmed

- Grated zest of 1 (organic) orange (see Note)

- 2 servings of pea protein powder or other protein base (see page 63)

- Handful of fresh spinach leaves, well washed

Place all ingredients in a blender. Blend for 3 to 5 minutes, until smooth. Serve cold, using a large-diameter glass or steel straw to drink.

Note

To make the zest, first wash the orange in warm soapy water and rinse well. Using a microplane or a box grater, grate the outer colorful portion of the peel. Stop grating when you start to reach the white pith beneath.

Roasted Strawberry Smoothie

PREP TIME: 5 MINUTES
MAKES 2 SERVINGS

Roasted strawberries? If you have not tried them, you may be in for a treat. Roasting the strawberries brings out a whole new dimension. To roast 1 pound of hulled fresh or thawed frozen strawberries, slice in half if large, spread on a baking sheet, and roast in a 350°F oven for 20 minutes. (You can roast the berries the night before making the smoothie, if you prefer.) The mesquite powder adds a rich, smoky flavor and more resistant starch to the mix.

- 1 cup purified water

- 1 cup ice cubes

- RS supplement (1 serving) or RS food ($1/4$ cup green banana flour, $1/2$ cup aquafaba, or others on page 64)

- Sweetener to taste (stevia, lo han)

- 1 cup roasted strawberries (see Headnote)

- 2 servings of pea protein powder or other protein base (see page 63)

- 1 teaspoon vanilla extract

- 1 tablespoon mesquite powder (optional)

Place all the ingredients in a blender. Blend for 3 to 5 minutes, until smooth. Serve cold, using a large-diameter glass or steel straw to drink.

Frozen Hot "Cocoa"

PREP TIME: 5 MINUTES

MAKES 2 SERVINGS

During the Reset you'll find that roasted carob makes a great caffeine-free, high RS stand-in for cocoa powder. When you use this recipe during the Maintenance phase, feel free to use carob or cocoa powder.

- $\frac{1}{2}$ cup old-fashioned (gluten-free) rolled oats

- 1 cup purified water

- 1 cup ice cubes

- RS supplement (1 serving) or RS food ($\frac{1}{4}$ cup green banana flour, $\frac{1}{2}$ cup aquafaba, or others on page 64)

- Sweetener to taste (stevia, lo han)

- 2 tablespoons toasted carob powder

- 2 servings of pea protein powder or other protein base (see page 63)

- $\frac{1}{2}$ frozen banana (organic, if with peel)

- 1 teaspoon vanilla extract

- Pinch of cayenne pepper (optional)

Add the oats to the blender and blend for 1 minute. Add the remaining ingredients and blend for 3 to 5 minutes, until smooth. Serve cold, using a large-diameter glass or steel straw to drink.

Classic Green Smoothie

PREP TIME: 5 MINUTES

MAKES 2 SERVINGS

This is fast and easy. You can use other mild greens, such as chard, romaine, kale, butter lettuce, or red leaf lettuce. Frozen greens work well also, but they are much more concentrated—you'll need only $\frac{1}{2}$ cup if using frozen.

- 1 cup purified water

- 1 cup ice cubes

- RS supplement (1 serving) or RS food ($\frac{1}{4}$ cup green banana flour, $\frac{1}{2}$ cup aquafaba, or others on page 64)

- Sweetener to taste (stevia, lo han)

- $\frac{1}{2}$ frozen banana (organic, if with peel)

- 2 servings of pea protein powder or other protein base (see page 63)

- 3 cups fresh spinach leaves, washed well

- 1 tablespoon chia seeds

- $\frac{1}{2}$ teaspoon minced fresh turmeric or ground turmeric

Place all the ingredients in a blender and blend for 3 to 5 minutes, until smooth. Serve cold, using a large-diameter glass or steel straw to drink.

Almond Crunch Oatmeal

PREP TIME: 5 MINUTES
MAKES 2 SERVINGS

Uncooked oats are rich in beta-glucans. These are unique polysaccharides that have been shown to improve the immune function, lower cholesterol, and improve cardiac health. When used uncooked, oats are also a rich source of resistant starch.

- $1/2$ cup old-fashioned (gluten-free) rolled oats
- 1 cup purified water
- 1 cup ice cubes
- RS supplement (1 serving) or RS food ($1/4$ cup green banana flour, $1/2$ cup aquafaba, or others on page 64)
- Sweetener to taste (stevia, lo han)
- $1/2$ teaspoon ground Ceylon cinnamon
- $1/8$ teaspoon ground cloves
- 2 servings of pea protein powder or other protein base (see page 63)
- 3 to 5 drops almond extract (optional)
- $1/4$ cup unsalted dry-roasted whole almonds

Place the oats in the blender and blend for 1 minute, until a powder. Add the water, ice, RS supplement, sweetener, cinnamon, cloves, protein powder, and almond extract, if using. Blend for 3 to 5 minutes, until smooth. Add the almonds and pulse for 10 to 20 seconds, just enough to break up the almonds and mix them in. Serve cold, using a large-diameter glass or steel straw to drink.

Papaya Ginger Mint

PREP TIME: 5 MINUTES

MAKES 2 SERVINGS

Papaya contains papain, a natural protein-digesting enzyme. The riper the papaya is, the less papain it contains, however, so avoid those that are overripe. This recipe also uses green banana flour. Most large natural foods supermarkets stock it; it has a pleasant banana flavor—less sweet than bananas and mildly tart. It has been popularized as an additional source of resistant starch. Also, this recipe works especially well with 1 cup of unsweetened nonfat Greek or Icelandic yogurt for the protein base.

- 1 cup purified water

- 1 cup ice cubes

- RS supplement (1 serving) or RS food ($1/4$ cup green banana flour, $1/2$ cup aquafaba, or others on page 64)

- Sweetener to taste (stevia, lo han)

- 1 cup frozen or fresh papaya (avoid overripe)

- 2 teaspoons grated fresh ginger

- Juice of $1/2$ lemon

- $1/4$ cup green banana flour, or $1/2$ frozen banana (organic, if with peel)

- 2 servings of pea protein powder or other protein base (see page 63)

- $1/4$ cup fresh mint leaves, and 2 sprigs for serving

- 1 tablespoon flax seeds

Place all the ingredients in the blender and blend for 3 to 5 minutes, until smooth. Garnish with a mint sprig. Serve cold, using a large-diameter glass or steel straw to drink.

Carrot Spice Cake

PREP TIME: 5 MINUTES

MAKES 2 SERVINGS

This recipe is a family favorite. My wife often juices a lot of carrots and has large amounts of pulp left over. If you ever find yourself in this situation, use twice as much carrot pulp as you would fresh carrot. If you have whole carrots in the refrigerator, they will work fine also; just chop them coarsely into 1- or 2-inch chunks so the blender can get a grip on them.

- 1 cup purified water
- 1 cup ice cubes
- RS supplement (1 serving) or RS food ($1/4$ cup green banana flour, $1/2$ cup aquafaba, or others on page 64)
- Sweetener to taste (stevia, lo han)
- $1/2$ frozen banana (organic, if with peel)
- 2 servings of pea protein powder or other protein base (see page 63)

- $1/2$ cup shredded carrot or baby carrots
- $1/2$ teaspoon vanilla extract
- $1/2$ teaspoon ground Ceylon cinnamon
- $1/8$ teaspoon ground nutmeg (preferably freshly grated)
- 1 tablespoon dried currants (optional)

Place all the ingredients except the currants in the blender and blend for 3 to 5 minutes, until smooth. Add the currants and pulse just a few times to mix them in. Serve cold, using a large-diameter glass or steel straw to drink.

Rosemary Pomegranate Blend

PREP TIME: 5 MINUTES
MAKES 2 SERVINGS

Legend has it that in the Middle Ages, if rosemary grew outside a home easily, it was a sign that the woman ruled the household. Our rosemary shrubs are out of control, so—my wife must be completely in charge! Culinary rosemary does differ from the ornamental variety. If you use ornamental rosemary, use about half as much and expect more of a pine flavor.

Rosemary has been shown to enhance cognitive function and protect brain cells against free radical stress. Pomegranate seeds have been proven to improve vascular health and benefit circulation. The fruits are seasonal and, to be candid, do take a lot of preparation. Thankfully, most natural foods supermarkets stock the frozen seeds.

- 1 cup purified water
- 1 cup ice cubes
- RS supplement (1 serving) or RS food ($^1/_4$ cup green banana flour, $^1/_2$ cup aquafaba, or others on page 64)
- Sweetener to taste (stevia, lo han)
- $^1/_2$ cup pomegranate seeds
- 2 servings of pea protein powder or other protein base (see page 63)
- 1 cup fresh spinach leaves, washed well
- 3 tablespoons chia seeds
- $^1/_2$ teaspoon minced fresh rosemary

Place all the ingredients in a blender and blend for 3 to 5 minutes, until smooth. Serve cold, using a large-diameter glass or steel straw to drink.

Apple Cinnamon Oatmeal

If you want a really efficient morning, try making this shake the night before. It is great however you make it, but it tastes even better when the apples and oats have more time to merge flavors.

- $1/2$ cup steel-cut oats or old-fashioned (gluten-free) rolled oats

- 1 cup purified water

- 1 cup ice cubes

- RS supplement (1 serving) or RS food ($1/4$ cup green banana flour, $1/2$ cup aquafaba, or others on page 64)

- Sweetener to taste (stevia, lo han)

- $1/2$ Granny Smith apple, cored

- 2 servings of pea protein powder or other protein base (see page 63)

- 2 tablespoons unsalted, dry-roasted whole almonds

- $1/2$ teaspoon ground Ceylon cinnamon

Place the oats in the blender and blend for 1 minute, until a powder. Add all the remaining ingredients and blend for 3 to 5 minutes, until smooth. Serve cold, using a large-diameter glass or steel straw to drink.

Carob, Pecan, and Banana

PREP TIME: 5 MINUTES

MAKES 2 SERVINGS

Pecans are rich in so many nutrients that they are practically a natural multivitamin. They can get rancid over time, however, so select pecan halves instead of pieces, and ideally buy in bulk, then store in the freezer, either raw or toasted.

Pecans are even more digestible and tastier when lightly toasted. To toast, spread the pecan halves out on a baking sheet and roast in a 250°F oven for 30 minutes.

- 1 cup purified water
- 1 cup ice cubes
- RS supplement (1 serving) or RS food ($1/4$ cup green banana flour, $1/2$ cup aquafaba, or others on page 64)
- Sweetener to taste (stevia, lo han)
- $1/2$ frozen banana (organic, if with peel)
- 2 servings of pea protein powder or other protein base (see page 63)
- 2 tablespoons toasted carob powder
- 2 tablespoons pecan halves or pieces

Place all the ingredients in the blender and blend for 3 to 5 minutes, until smooth. Serve cold, using a large-diameter glass or steel straw to drink.

Super Red Blend

PREP TIME: 5 MINUTES
MAKES 2 SERVINGS

Guaranteed to stain your shirt, this mixture is rich in betaine and polyphenols. I usually use raw beets. Just trim the tips, save the stems and leaves for another use, and give the bulbs a thorough scrub with a coarse brush.

- 1 cup purified water
- 1 cup ice cubes
- RS supplement (1 serving) or RS food ($1/4$ cup green banana flour, $1/2$ cup aquafaba, or others on page 64)
- Sweetener to taste (stevia, lo han)
- $1/2$ cup chopped blanched or raw beets
- $1/4$ cup frozen pitted dark cherries
- $1/4$ cup frozen pomegranate seeds
- 2 servings of pea protein powder or other protein base (see page 63)
- 1 tablespoon hemp seeds
- $1/2$ teaspoon minced fresh turmeric or ground turmeric

Place all the ingredients in a blender and blend for 3 to 5 minutes, until smooth. Serve cold, using a large-diameter glass or steel straw to drink.

Banana Pumpkin Pie

PREP TIME: 5 MINUTES

MAKES 2 SERVINGS

Here is a great use for any extra pumpkin from the holidays. If you have not yet tried banana peels, this is a great shake to see what you think. They help round out the flavor and also add texture.

- 1 cup purified water
- 1 cup ice cubes
- RS supplement (1 serving) or RS food ($1/4$ cup green banana flour, $1/2$ cup aquafaba, or others on page 64)
- Sweetener to taste (stevia, lo han)
- $1/2$ frozen (organic) banana, with peel
- $1/2$ cup canned pumpkin
- 2 servings of pea protein powder or other protein base (see page 63)
- $1/2$ teaspoon vanilla extract
- $1/4$ teaspoon pumpkin pie spice

Place all the ingredients in a blender and blend for 3 to 5 minutes, until smooth. Serve cold, using a large-diameter glass or steel straw to drink.

Green Pina Colada

PREP TIME: 5 MINUTES

MAKES 2 SERVINGS

This smoothie is a flavor classic. Skip the rum during your Reset, okay? You may need less sweetener than other shake recipes, owing to the pineapple. I prefer frozen pineapple chunks, but look for ones with no added sugar. If fresh pineapple is on sale, it is usually in season and a pineapple has so much fruit that it's worth buying fresh and freezing some of it.

- 1 cup purified water

- 1 cup ice cubes

- RS supplement (1 serving) or RS food ($1/4$ cup green banana flour, $1/2$ cup aquafaba, or others on page 64)

- Sweetener to taste (stevia, lo han)

- $1/2$ frozen banana (organic, if with peel)

- $1/4$ cup pineapple chunks

- 2 servings of pea protein powder or other protein base (see page 63)

- 2 cups fresh spinach leaves, washed well

- 2 tablespoons fresh coconut meat or unsweetened dried coconut

- $1/2$ teaspoon minced fresh ginger or ground ginger

Place all the ingredients in the blender and blend for 3 to 5 minutes, until smooth. Serve cold, using a large-diameter glass or steel straw to drink.

Carob Mint

PREP TIME: 5 MINUTES
MAKES 2 SERVINGS

Here is a great flavor combo. You can also use a drop of food-grade essential oil of peppermint, if you do not have any mint leaves handy.

- 1 cup purified water

- 1 cup ice cubes

- RS supplement (1 serving) or RS food ($\frac{1}{4}$ cup green banana flour, $\frac{1}{2}$ cup aquafaba, or others on page 64)

- Sweetener to taste (stevia, lo han)

- $\frac{1}{2}$ frozen banana (organic, if with peel)

- 1 tablespoon toasted carob powder

- 2 tablespoons chopped fresh mint

- 2 servings of pea protein powder or other protein base (see page 63)

- 2 tablespoons walnut halves or pieces

Place all the ingredients in the blender and blend for 3 to 5 minutes, until smooth. Serve cold, using a large-diameter glass or steel straw to drink.

Macadamia Green Tea

PREP TIME: 5 MINUTES

MAKES 2 SERVINGS

In Western cultures, we see tea as a beverage; Eastern cultures use its delicate flavor also for desserts and savory dishes. During the Reset phase, you can get the flavor of green tea by using decaffeinated green tea leaves. Look for a decaf product made with the CO_2 process, as opposed to solvent extraction. During the Maintenance phase, $1/2$ teaspoon of matcha powder works well in this shake, assuming you are not caffeine sensitive.

- 1 cup purified water
- 1 cup ice cubes
- RS supplement (1 serving) or RS food ($1/4$ cup green banana flour, $1/2$ cup aquafaba, or others on page 64)
- Sweetener to taste (stevia, lo han)
- $1/2$ frozen banana (organic, if with peel)
- 2 servings of pea protein powder or other protein base (see page 63)
- $1/3$ cup macadamia nuts
- 1 bag decaffeinated green tea

Place all the ingredients in a blender, emptying the contents of the tea bag into the blender as well. Blend for 3 to 5 minutes, until smooth. Serve cold, using a large-diameter glass or steel straw to drink.

Blueberry Cheesecake

PREP TIME: 5 MINUTES

MAKES 2 SERVINGS

To get the texture right, this shake is especially good when made the night before, or at least an hour in advance. If you are not dairy sensitive, try using cottage cheese as the protein base.

- 1 cup purified water

- 1 cup ice cubes

- RS supplement (1 serving) or RS food ($1/4$ cup green banana flour, $1/2$ cup aquafaba, or others on page 64)

- Sweetener to taste (stevia, lo han)

- $1/2$ cup frozen blueberries

- 2 servings of pea protein powder or other protein base (see page 63)

- $1/4$ cup chia seeds

- Juice of 1 lemon

Place all the ingredients in the blender and blend for 3 to 5 minutes, until smooth. Serve cold, using a large-diameter glass or steel straw to drink.

Green Plum Cooler

PREP TIME: 5 MINUTES
MAKES 2 SERVINGS

I love fresh plums, but it seems they have a narrow window of perfect ripeness. Using them in shakes spreads the season a bit because you can use them even if they are under- or overripe. The "green" in the recipe title here refers to the color of the final product, as the plums do not have to be green—black, red, or green, or pluots, all work fine. You can even use 2 dried prunes as a substitute for each plum.

- 1 cup purified water
- 1 cup ice cubes
- RS supplement (1 serving) or RS food ($1/4$ cup green banana flour, $1/2$ cup aquafaba, or others on page 64)
- Sweetener to taste (stevia, lo han)
- 2 ripe plums, pitted
- Juice of 1 lemon
- 2 servings of pea protein powder or other protein base (see page 63)
- $1/4$ cup fresh parsley

Place all the ingredients in the blender and blend for 3 to 5 minutes, until smooth. Serve cold, using a large-diameter glass or steel straw to drink.

Orange Kiwi Cilantro

PREP TIME: 5 MINUTES
MAKES 2 SERVINGS

Like all greens, cilantro has some powerful detox properties, but it may be one of the best. Cilantro is the term we use for the leaves of the same plant that produces coriander seeds. Unfortunately, about 15 percent of people have a gene combination that can make cilantro taste like soap, even though that's not the case for the seeds. Whenever you make this shake for friends or guests, ask ahead how they feel about cilantro. For those who hate it, even the tiny bit in this shake can ruin the experience for them.

- 1 cup purified water
- 1 cup ice cubes
- RS supplement (1 serving) or RS food ($1/4$ cup green banana flour, $1/2$ cup aquafaba, or others on page 64)
- 1 tablespoon green banana flour
- Sweetener to taste (stevia, lo han)

- 1 orange, peeled with some white pith retained
- 1 kiwi, peeled
- 2 servings of pea protein powder or other protein base (see page 63)
- $1/3$ cup fresh cilantro
- 2 tablespoons sunflower seeds
- $1/2$ teaspoon minced fresh ginger or ground ginger

Place all the ingredients in the blender and blend for 3 to 5 minutes, until smooth. Serve cold, using a large-diameter glass or steel straw to drink.

Peach and Rosewater

PREP TIME: 5 MINUTES
MAKES 2 SERVINGS

You can usually find rosewater in larger grocery stores or in East Indian or Middle Eastern grocers. It is worth finding, since it lends a flavor all on its own. Food-grade essential oil of rose can work, but it is so easy to use too much. If you're using the essential oil, dip the tip of a toothpick in the oil and then pour water over the toothpick into the blender.

- $1/2$ cup purified water
- $1/2$ cup rosewater
- 1 cup ice cubes
- RS supplement (1 serving) or RS food ($1/4$ cup green banana flour, $1/2$ cup aquafaba, or others on page 64)

- Sweetener to taste (stevia, lo han)
- 1 ripe peach, pitted
- 2 servings of pea protein powder or other protein base (see page 63)
- 2 tablespoons white sesame seeds

Place all the ingredients in the blender and blend for 3 to 5 minutes, until smooth. Serve cold, using a large-diameter glass or steel straw to drink.

Plum Lime Cooler

PREP TIME: 5 MINUTES
MAKES 2 SERVINGS

Here is another good use of fresh plums. They contain a natural gentle laxative called dihydroxyphenyl isatin, which helps prevent reabsorption of bile from the liver. This recipe also includes fennel seeds; if you are prone to gas or bloating, see if fennel reduces your symptoms. It gives the mixture a subtle licorice/anise flavor, but if you hate this taste, it works fine without it.

- 1 cup purified water
- 1 cup ice cubes
- RS supplement (1 serving) or RS food ($1/4$ cup green banana flour, $1/2$ cup aquafaba, or others on page 64)
- 1 tablespoon green banana flour
- Sweetener to taste (stevia, lo han)
- 1 ripe plum, pitted
- Juice of 1 lime
- 2 servings of pea protein powder or other protein base (see page 63)
- 1 teaspoon fennel seeds (optional)

Place all the ingredients in the blender and blend for 3 to 5 minutes, until smooth. Serve cold, using a large-diameter glass or steel straw to drink.

Blackberry Almond Chia

PREP TIME: 5 MINUTES
MAKES 2 SERVINGS

Like several recipes in this book, this one benefits from a bit of almond extract. A friend asked me why I do not specify natural almond extract. Here's the short answer: it does not matter. The pure almond flavor in almonds comes from a compound called benzaldehyde, and benzaldehyde is most concentrated in bitter almonds. (It is also found in small amounts in various other plants like cinnamon.) Most natural almond extract is extracted from those bitter almonds. The concern is that the extraction process inevitably leaves a touch of cyanide in the final product. In fact, if you consumed several bottles of natural almond extract at once, it could be harmful. Synthetic almond extract also gets its flavor from benzaldehyde, minus the cyanide.

Which is better? Benzaldehyde in the amounts found in almonds or almond extracts is completely harmless. So are both synthetic and natural almond extract. You may find a natural almond extract with fewer other chemicals or preservatives, but otherwise both taste the same and both are nontoxic. (If you think someone in your home may drink it in ridiculous quantities, synthetic almond extract would be safer.)

If you're on the Reset, omit the aquafaba and sweetener in this recipe.

- 1 cup purified water
- 1 cup ice cubes
- RS supplement (1 serving) or RS food ($\frac{1}{4}$ cup green banana flour, $\frac{1}{2}$ cup aquafaba, or others on page 64)
- Sweetener to taste (stevia, lo han)

- 1 cup fresh or frozen blackberries
- $\frac{1}{4}$ cup chia seeds
- 2 servings of pea protein powder or other protein base (see page 63)
- $\frac{1}{2}$ teaspoon almond extract

Place all the ingredients in the blender and blend for 3 to 5 minutes, until smooth. Serve cold, using a large-diameter glass or steel straw to drink.

Blueberry Lime Smoothie

PREP TIME: 5 MINUTES
MAKES 2 SERVINGS

This shake can also be made with almost any other type of berry, if you do not happen to have blueberries on hand. The final pinch of sea salt is a nice touch, so be sure not to forget it.

- 1 cup purified water
- 1 cup ice cubes
- RS supplement (1 serving) or RS food ($1/4$ cup green banana flour, $1/2$ cup aquafaba, or others on page 64)
- 1 cup frozen blueberries
- Juice of 2 limes
- Grated zest of 1 lime
- Sweetener to taste (stevia, lo han)
- 2 servings of pea protein powder or other protein base (see page 63)
- 2 tablespoons chia seeds
- $1/2$ teaspoon vanilla extract
- Pinch of coarse sea salt

Add all the ingredients except the salt to the blender and blend for 3 to 5 minutes, until smooth. Pour into serving glasses and sprinkle the salt on top. Serve cold, using a large-diameter glass or steel straw. Use the straw to lightly stir in the salt.

Blood Orange Sunflower Smoothie

PREP TIME: 5 MINUTES
MAKES 2 SERVINGS

It is often the case that more pigmented varieties of a food are richer in protective phytonutrients. This rule holds true for blood oranges as well. One study using mice showed that blood oranges had specific effects in reducing steatohepatitis, the fat clogging the liver. Expect blood oranges to have a rich orange taste with undertones of raspberry. It is also normal that they are more resistant to peeling. As with all citrus, try to leave some of the white pith on, as it is the main source of powerful bioflavonoids like hesperidin methyl chalcone, which improve liver health and vascular integrity.

For this recipe, try toasting the sunflower seeds. Buy them raw and spread out on a baking sheet, then roast in a 225°F oven for 20 minutes. Store in the freezer in an airtight glass container.

- 1 cup purified water

- 1 cup ice cubes

- RS supplement (1 serving) or RS food ($1/4$ cup green banana flour, $1/2$ cup aquafaba, or others on page 64)

- 1 blood orange, peeled with some white pith retained

- Sweetener to taste (stevia, lo han)

- 2 servings of pea protein powder or other protein base (see page 63)

- 2 tablespoons sunflower seeds, preferably toasted

- $1/4$ teaspoon minced fresh ginger or ground ginger

Place all the ingredients in the blender and blend for 3 to 5 minutes, until smooth. Serve cold, using a large-diameter glass or steel straw to drink.

Black Forest Cherry Smoothie

PREP TIME: 5 MINUTES

MAKES 2 SERVINGS

Remember the rule: foods that stain are good for you. When it comes to your metabolism, staining is good, and staining red is especially good. Studies have shown that the anthocyanins in cherries make the liver more able to tap into stored triglycerides and eliminate the buildup of uric acid that often leads to joint pain.

- 1 cup purified water
- 1 cup ice cubes
- RS supplement (1 serving) or RS food ($1/4$ cup green banana flour, $1/2$ cup aquafaba, or others on page 64)
- Sweetener to taste (stevia, lo han)
- $1/2$ (organic) frozen banana, with peel

- $1/2$ cup frozen pitted dark cherries
- 2 tablespoons roasted carob powder
- 2 servings of pea protein powder or other protein base (see page 63)
- 1 cup fresh spinach leaves, well washed

Place all the ingredients in the blender and blend for 3 to 5 minutes, until smooth. Serve cold, using a large-diameter glass or steel straw to drink.

Green Power Smoothie

PREP TIME: 5 MINUTES

MAKES 2 SERVINGS

Is it possible to eat too many greens? It is possible, but not a probable risk for the vast majority of us. Chlorophyll has unparalleled effects when it comes to preventing toxicants from recirculating from the intestinal tract back into the bloodstream. This mix is a tasty way to get more greens. Many supermarkets offer "power greens," which are a blend of several types of washed and trimmed greens. If you cannot find such a blend, try combining spinach, chard, and kale, or just use spinach by itself.

- 1 cup purified water

- 1 cup ice cubes

- RS supplement (1 serving) or RS food ($1/4$ cup green banana flour, $1/2$ cup aquafaba, or others on page 64)

- $1/2$ frozen banana (organic, if with peel)

- Sweetener to taste (stevia, lo han)

- $1/2$ medium avocado, peeled and seeded

- 3 cups greens blend (spinach, chard, kale)

- 2 servings of pea protein powder or other protein base (see page 63)

- $1/3$ cup fresh parsley

Place all the ingredients in the blender and blend for 3 to 5 minutes, until smooth. Serve cold, using a large-diameter glass or steel straw to drink.

Raspberry Tigernut Blast

PREP TIME: 5 MINUTES
MAKES 2 SERVINGS

Tigernuts are not nuts in the botanical sense. It would be more accurate to think of them as tiny dried potatoes. They are rich in resistant starch, many other forms of fiber, and minerals such as zinc and manganese. Tigernuts are the swollen roots, or tubers, of many varieties of wild grasses. Scientists now think that such tubers made up a large portion of the diet of early human beings.

You can find tigernuts with and without the skin—either will taste fine, although the skin provides more fiber. If you eat them as a snack, soaking them first is not mandatory, but will make them easier to chew. For use in this shake, soaking is unnecessary if your blender is a strong one.

- $1/2$ cup tigernuts
- 1 cup purified water
- 1 cup ice cubes
- RS supplement (1 serving) or RS food ($1/4$ cup green banana flour, $1/2$ cup aquafaba, or others on page 64)
- 1 tablespoon green banana flour
- Sweetener to taste (stevia, lo han)
- 1 cup fresh or frozen raspberries
- 2 servings of pea protein powder or other protein base (see page 63)

Place the tigernuts in the blender and blend for 2 minutes, until a powder forms. Add the remaining ingredients and blend for 3 to 5 minutes, until smooth. Serve cold, using a large-diameter glass or steel straw to drink.

Peppermint Brazil Nut Smoothie

PREP TIME: 5 MINUTES

MAKES 2 SERVINGS

Brazil nuts are the nonpareil food source of selenium, although the exact amount per nut can vary from as low as 30 mcg to as high as 110 mcg. You can consider 1 or 2 Brazil nuts per day as a simple insurance policy on top of your diet and supplementation.

- 1 cup purified water

- 1 cup ice cubes

- RS supplement (1 serving) or RS food ($1/4$ cup green banana flour, $1/2$ cup aquafaba, or others on page 64)

- $1/2$ (organic) frozen banana, with peel

- Sweetener to taste (stevia, lo han)

- 2 Brazil nuts

- 1 to 3 drops food-grade peppermint essential oil

- 2 servings of pea protein powder or other protein base (see page 63)

Place all the ingredients in the blender and blend for 3 to 5 minutes, until smooth. Serve cold, using a large-diameter glass or steel straw to drink.

Walnut Carob Brownie

PREP TIME: 5 MINUTES
MAKES 2 SERVINGS

Trust me on this. As long as they are unsalted, the black beans do not impart any specific flavor, but they do a great job providing the brownie texture and color. They are one of the richest of all sources of fiber and bioflavonoids.

- 1 cup purified water

- 1 cup ice cubes

- RS supplement (1 serving) or RS food ($1/4$ cup green banana flour, $1/2$ cup aquafaba, or others on page 64)

- $1/2$ cup unsalted canned or cooked black beans, drained and rinsed

- $1/2$ (organic) frozen banana, with peel

- Sweetener to taste (stevia, lo han)

- 2 tablespoons roasted carob powder

- 2 servings of pea protein powder or other protein base (see page 63)

- $1/2$ cup walnut halves

Place all the ingredients in the blender and blend for 3 to 5 minutes, until smooth. Serve cold, using a large-diameter glass or steel straw to drink.

Lemon Basil Smoothie

PREP TIME: 5 MINUTES

MAKES 2 SERVINGS

You cannot go wrong with basil. It is a powerful adaptogen and nervine. Effective at alleviating the effects of chronic stress, it is also a good antiviral immune tonic. Whenever you feel like you are on the edge of a cold, make this shake and also make some pesto for dinner.

- 1 cup purified water
- 1 cup ice cubes
- RS supplement (1 serving) or RS food ($1/4$ cup green banana flour, $1/2$ cup aquafaba, or others on page 64)
- $1/2$ (organic) frozen banana, with peel
- Sweetener to taste (stevia, lo han)
- 8 fresh basil leaves
- Juice of 1 lemon

Place all the ingredients in the blender and blend for 3 to 5 minutes, until smooth. Serve cold, using a large-diameter glass or steel straw to drink.

Cardamom Peach

PREP TIME: 5 MINUTES
MAKES 2 SERVINGS

Like other stone fruits, fresh peaches have a narrow window of optimal ripeness. Buy them frozen or freeze your own, if you have an abundance of them. Cardamom is almost always a perfect pairing with peaches. It is a spice used extensively in East Indian cuisine, but often ignored elsewhere. Cardamom is a specific remedy in Ayurveda medicine for breaking down deposits of bile and fat that are trapped in the liver. Ground cardamom seed will work, but the pods, with their seeds, will often have a fresher flavor.

- 1 cup purified water
- 1 cup ice cubes
- RS supplement (1 serving) or RS food ($1/4$ cup green banana flour, $1/2$ cup aquafaba, or others on page 64)
- 1 ripe peach, pitted
- Sweetener to taste (stevia, lo han)
- $1/2$ teaspoon seeds from cardamom pods
- 2 tablespoons chia seeds

Place all the ingredients in a blender and blend for 3 to 5 minutes, until smooth. Serve cold, using a large-diameter glass or steel straw to drink.

chapter eight

Dinner and Unlimited Food Recipes

QUICK BOWLS

Bowls have to be one of the most versatile dishes out there. Not only can you include as much as you like, portion-wise, but you can fill a bowl with all sorts of delicious ingredients. You might like more vegetables, or you might like more rice—either way, there really is no wrong way to make this great dinner favorite!

10-Minute Grilled Salmon Bowl

PREP TIME: 35 MINUTES (INCLUDES COOKING THE BROWN RICE)
COOK TIME: 10 MINUTES
SERVES 1

Fish that is cooked too long can take on a rubbery texture. The secret to cooking this salmon is to undercook it slightly. This way, it can continue to "cook" as it rests off the heat awaiting assembly in the bowl.

- Avocado oil cooking spray
- 1 tablespoon whole-grain Dijon mustard
- Juice of $1/2$ lemon
- 2 garlic cloves, crushed

- 1 (4- to 6-ounce) salmon fillet
- $1/2$ to $3/4$ cup cooked brown rice, warm
- Salt and pepper

OPTIONAL TOPPINGS

- Sliced radish
- Fresh baby spinach
- Sliced cucumber
- Sliced carrot

- Sliced scallions
- Sprouts
- $1/3$ avocado, sliced

Lightly coat a skillet with the avocado oil cooking spray and place the pan over medium heat.

Combine the mustard, lemon juice, and garlic in a bowl and spread the paste on the salmon fillet.

Place the salmon in the pan skin side up and cook for 3 to 7 minutes (depending on thickness), then turn over, adding a bit more cooking spray to the pan if necessary, and cook an additional 2 to 5 minutes, or until firm and nearly cooked through.

Place the warm rice in the serving bowl and top with the salmon. Add as many optional toppings as desired. Season to taste with salt and pepper, and enjoy.

Vegan version

Instead of salmon, consider using Quorn brand meatless and soy-free chicken cutlets or organic non-GMO extra-firm tofu. You also have the option to drink an extra serving of protein powder with dinner instead.

Asian Chicken Bowl

PREP TIME: 35 MINUTES (INCLUDES COOKING THE BROWN RICE)
COOK TIME: 10 TO 15 MINUTES
SERVES 1

This recipe utilizes a few basic ingredients and brings them together for a quick, easy, and delicious meal. All it takes is a fistful of chicken, seasonings, and some delicious veggies like bok choy. In a rush? Have the brown rice ready to go and it'll take you only about 10 minutes.

- Avocado oil cooking spray
- 1 or 2 garlic cloves
- 1 teaspoon shredded fresh ginger
- 3 or 4 stems and leaves of bok choy, separated and chopped
- 1 8-ounce package sliced white button mushrooms
- 1 cup chopped cooked chicken
- 1 tablespoon soy sauce
- $1/2$ teaspoon onion powder
- $1/2$ to $3/4$ cup cooked brown rice, warm
- 1 or 2 green onions, chopped
- $3/4$ cup chopped or shredded raw carrot
- $1 1/2$ tablespoons chopped cashews
- Salt and pepper

Lightly coat a wide skillet or wok with the cooking spray and warm the pan over medium-high heat.

Add the garlic and ginger, and sauté for 30 to 60 seconds, until softened. Add the bok choy stems and the mushrooms, and cook until the stems are soft, about 2 minutes. Add the leaves and continue to cook until the mushrooms are browned, about 3 minutes more.

Coat another skillet with some cooking spray, then add the chicken, soy sauce, and onion powder. Stir the ingredients until cooked, about 5 minutes (or until warmed, if using shredded chicken).

Place the brown rice, bok choy, and chicken into a serving bowl and top with the green onions, carrot, and cashews. Season to taste with salt and pepper.

Vegan version

Instead of the chicken, feel free to use tempeh, tofu, or edamame, using organic and non-GMO products. Other possibilities include spirulina or nutritional yeast. You also have the option to drink an extra serving of protein powder with dinner instead.

Sprouted-Almond Fish "Taco" Bowl

PREP TIME: 5 MINUTES
COOK TIME: 10 MINUTES
SERVES 1

Fresh, simply flavored, and classic Mexican. This isn't the kind of Mexican food you'll find at fast-food restaurants; you'll find it's light and different, yet filling. The sprouted almonds add a nice touch.

- Avocado oil cooking spray
- 1 cup sprouted almonds, crushed
- 1 lime
- 1 (4- to 6-ounce) fillet of white fish of choice
- 1/2 cup canned or cooked pinto beans, drained and rinsed
- 2 cups shredded lettuce
- 1 small onion, chopped
- 1 ripe medium tomato, cut into 1/2-inch slices
- 2 rice tortillas, torn into small pieces
- Salt and pepper
- Chopped fresh cilantro (optional)

Lightly coat a skillet with some of the cooking spray and place the pan over medium-high heat. Spread the almonds on a plate.

Squeeze about half the lime juice onto the fish, rubbing it in, then dredge in the almonds. Place the fish in the hot pan and sauté for 3 to 5 minutes. Turn the fish over, add a little more cooking spray to the pan, and cook an additional 3 to 5 minutes or until the fish is firm and flakes easily.

Place the beans, lettuce, and onion in a serving bowl. Add the tomato, then flake the fish with a fork and add to the bowl. Sprinkle the rice tortillas over the top. Squeeze the remaining lime juice over, season to taste with salt and pepper, and top with the cilantro, if using.

Vegan version

Instead of the fish, feel free to use organic and non-GMO firm tofu. You also have the option to drink an extra serving of protein powder with dinner instead.

LIGHT DISHES

Chicken and Apple Tomato Salad

PREP TIME: 10 MINUTES

SERVES 2

This recipe might seem a little out of the ordinary at first. It uses sliced tomatoes as a base for this fantastic chicken and apple salad. It offers a burst of flavor that makes your mid-day meal a little special. If you're choosing the yogurt option, add some healthy fat to the mixture, like a side of 8 almonds or $1/3$ avocado.

- 2 cups diced cooked chicken
- 1 small apple, cored and diced
- 2 green onions, diced
- Chopped cilantro, plus more to serve (optional)
- 2 tablespoons egg-free mayonnaise or fat-free, high-protein plain yogurt
- 2 ripe tomatoes, cut into $1/2$-inch slices
- Salt and pepper

Mix the chicken, apple, green onions, and cilantro, if using, in a bowl. Add the mayonnaise and stir to coat well.

Place the tomato slices on individual plates and spoon some salad on top. Sprinkle with salt and pepper to taste. If desired, sprinkle a little more cilantro on top.

Vegan version

Instead of the chicken, feel free to use Quorn brand meatless and soy-free chicken tenders or unseasoned organic and non-GMO tempeh. Also, use a vegan alternative to mayonnaise, like the Veganaise brand spread. You also have the option to drink an extra serving of protein powder with dinner instead.

Leftovers

If you find yourself with extra chicken salad, cover with wrap and refrigerate for lunch the next day—all you'll need is another tomato.

Quinoa Lettuce Wraps

PREP TIME: 10 MINUTES
COOK TIME: 15 MINUTES
SERVES 4

Does your family celebrate Taco Tuesdays? It's one of the best days in our household, and we just love the opportunity to get creative and enjoy all those Latin flavors. These tacos, in particular, are great because they contain good sources of both protein and fiber. The freshness is perfect for summer, but it honestly makes for a great meal all year long.

- 1 cup quinoa, rinsed
- 2 tablespoons avocado oil
- 3 garlic cloves, minced
- $1/2$ red onion, thinly sliced
- Pinch of sea salt
- Freshly ground pepper
- 1 (15-ounce) can black beans, drained and rinsed
- 1 cup drained canned or thawed frozen (organic) corn kernels

- 1 cup thinly sliced red bell pepper
- 2 cups shredded cooked (organic) chicken
- 2 tablespoons (MSG-free) taco seasoning
- Juice of 1 lime
- Juice of 1 lemon
- $1/3$ cup chopped fresh cilantro
- 1 teaspoon freshly ground cumin seeds (or ground cumin)
- 1 head butter lettuce, leaves separated and washed well

OPTIONAL

- $1/2$ cup chopped fresh cilantro
- $1/2$ cup sliced jalapeño
- 2 Roma (plum) tomatoes, diced

- 1 medium avocado, diced
- 1 (4-ounce) can green chiles

Cook the quinoa according to the package directions.

Meanwhile, place the avocado oil, garlic, red onion, salt, and pepper in a large skillet over medium heat. Cook for 8 minutes, or until fragrant.

Add the quinoa, beans, corn, bell pepper, and chicken, stirring until warm. Stir in the taco seasoning, and the lime and lemon juices. Sprinkle with the cilantro and cumin.

Take each lettuce leaf and dollop some of the quinoa mixture in the center. Fill with the optional garnishes, and fold the edges of the leaf onto themselves to form a wrap. Serve at once.

Vegan version

Instead of the chicken, feel free to use non-GMO tempeh. You also have the option to drink an extra serving of protein powder with dinner instead.

Leftovers

If you have any quinoa mixture left, wrap it tightly and refrigerate to enjoy some more tacos tomorrow.

Healthy Turkey Lettuce Wraps

PREP TIME: 5 MINUTES
COOK TIME: 15 MINUTES
MAKES 12 TO 16 LETTUCE WRAPS, OR 4 SERVINGS

Lettuce wraps are a great way to get good protein while enjoying a light and quick meal. Remember, when you're eating healthy, there are ways to alter those earlier, favorite "comfort" foods to suit the diet and make them even more enjoyable. Just add cooked rice! When dividing the mixture among the lettuce wraps, ensure that you have a 1:1 ratio of turkey to rice. This results in the right crunch and combination of flavors.

FOR THE SAUCE

- $^2/_3$ cup Eden gluten-free teriyaki sauce
- $^2/_3$ cup water
- 1 tablespoon xylitol
- $^1/_2$ teaspoon dry mustard
- $^1/_2$ teaspoon granulated garlic
- $^1/_2$ teaspoon onion powder
- $^1/_4$ teaspoon ground ginger
- $1^1/_2$ tablespoons sweet chili sauce

FOR THE WRAPS

- 1 tablespoon avocado oil
- 1 cup finely chopped carrots (about 2 medium)
- 1 cup chopped celery (about 1 stalk)
- 1 cup chopped white button mushrooms
- Sea salt and pepper
- 1 pound (organic) lean ground turkey
- 3 green onions
- 2 cups cooked brown rice
- 12 to 16 butter or iceberg lettuce leaves (have extra because some may tear)

MAKE THE SAUCE Combine all the ingredients in a small saucepan and heat over medium heat until the mixture comes to a low boil. Stir constantly for 4 minutes to thicken. Remove from the heat.

PREPARE THE WRAPS Heat the oil in a large saucepan or skillet over medium-high heat. When hot enough that a drop of water sizzles, add the carrots, celery, and mushrooms. Stir to coat with the oil, and lightly season with salt and pepper. Sauté the vegetables, stirring occasionally, for 6 minutes or until tender.

Add the turkey to the pan, breaking it up with a spatula as it cooks. Lightly season again with salt and pepper, then add the green onions and cook for 5 to 6 minutes, or until the turkey is cooked.

Drain any liquid from the turkey in the pan and then spoon about $1/2$ cup of the sauce over. Stir to coat the mixture, and add additional sauce as desired.

Lay the lettuce leaves out on the counter and spread with the rice, then spoon on some turkey. Fold and serve with remaining sauce on the side.

Vegan version

Instead of turkey, feel free to use crumbled organic non-GMO tempeh. You also have the option to drink an extra serving of protein powder with dinner instead.

Leftovers

Save any leftover turkey mixture separately, covered and refrigerated, to be put into new lettuce wraps the next day.

Pumpkin Salad

PREP TIME: 10 MINUTES
COOK TIME: 30 MINUTES
SERVES 1

Whether you need an easy prep recipe or something quick, this pumpkin salad has the answer. Best of all, you can also replace the pumpkin with butternut squash, depending on the season, so you can enjoy this recipe all year long.

- 2 teaspoons avocado oil
- 5 cups diced pumpkin or butternut squash
- Salt and pepper
- 2 tablespoons fresh orange juice
- 1 1/2 tablespoons macadamia nut oil or grapeseed oil
- 1 1/2 teaspoons lemon juice
- 1/2 cup chopped walnuts
- 8 cups lightly packed arugula
- 1/2 cup fresh blueberries or raspberries
- 2 skinless, boneless chicken breasts, cooked, cooled, and shredded

Preheat the oven to 450°F.

In a bowl, toss the pumpkin cubes with the avocado oil, and add salt and pepper to taste. Spread the pumpkin on a baking sheet and roast for 15 minutes. Turn the cubes over and continue to roast for another 15 minutes, until soft and lightly browned.

Let the pumpkin cool. Meanwhile, whisk the orange juice, macadamia nut oil, and lemon juice in a large bowl. Add the walnuts and arugula, stirring to coat with the vinaigrette. Season again with salt and pepper.

Add the berries, chicken, and pumpkin, and toss gently. Serve at once.

Vegan version

Instead of chicken, feel free to use Quorn meatless and soy-free chicken cutlets. You also have the option to drink an extra serving of protein powder with dinner instead.

Yummy Salad Jar

PREP TIME: 10 MINUTES

SERVES 1

A salad jar is simple, healthy, and delicious—it even looks amazing! It makes for the perfect meal because you can assemble it quickly and be out the door in a hurry. The best part? The jar is a ready-made serving portion. And feel free to get creative! If you want to use rice or potatoes instead of chickpeas, go for it! Play with the ingredients but have them be as colorful as possible.

- 2 tablespoons dressing of choice
- 1 mason jar
- 1 pint grape or cherry tomatoes
- $1/2$ cup cooked or canned chickpeas, drained and rinsed
- 1 roasted red bell pepper, cored and seeded
- 2 or 3 small pitted olives
- 2 ounces arugula, washed and dried
- 2 ounces fresh spinach, washed and dried
- 1 cup shredded cooked chicken
- 3 or 4 walnuts, chopped

Pour the dressing into the bottom of the mason jar. Stack the ingredients on top, as follows: tomatoes, chickpeas, roasted red pepper, olives, arugula, spinach, chicken, and walnuts. (Alternatively, package the dressing in a small container to carry along and add when you're ready to eat.) Ideally, the salad jar can last 3 or 4 days, but eating it within 1 or 2 days is optimal.

Vegan version

Instead of the chicken, feel free to use Quorn meatless and soy-free chicken cutlets or organic non-GMO extra-firm tofu. You also have the option to drink an extra serving of protein powder with dinner instead.

Cold Potato, Beet, Carrot, and Pea Salad with Dill

PREP TIME: 10 MINUTES
COOK TIME: 45 MINUTES
SERVES 2

This is a salad for those who march to the "beet" of their own drum. It's filled with all sorts of great vegetables, and is an easy way to put together a meal without ever having to turn on your oven. The addition of dill adds a nice kick, too. You can prepare the beets, potatoes, and carrots ahead of time; and since the salad is served cold, it's ready to go.

- 2 medium red or golden beets, tops trimmed
- 3 medium Yukon Gold potatoes
- 2 medium carrots, cut into $1/2$-inch pieces
- 1 cup coarsely chopped red onion
- $1/2$ cup chopped natural dill pickles, such as Bubbies
- $1/4$ cup chopped fresh dill
- $1/4$ cup macadamia nut oil or grapeseed oil
- $1/4$ cup red wine vinegar
- 2 teaspoons whole-grain Dijon mustard
- $1/2$ teaspoon coarse sea salt
- $1/4$ teaspoon freshly ground black pepper
- $1/2$ cup thawed frozen petite green peas
- 1 (3.75-ounce) can sardines, drained

Halve the beets and place them in a vegetable steamer over boiling water. Steam, covered, until tender when pierced with the tip of a knife, 20 to 35 minutes depending on the size. Let cool. Use a paring knife to slip off the skin, snip the root, and then cut the beets into $1/2$-inch cubes.

Meanwhile, place the potatoes in a saucepan and cover with water. Bring to a boil, and cook, covered, until almost tender, 15 minutes. Add the carrots and cook about 5 minutes more, until the potatoes are tender and the carrots are crisp-tender. Drain and let cool. Using a paring knife, peel the loosened skins from the potatoes and cut into $1/2$-inch cubes.

In a large bowl, combine the beets, potatoes, carrots, the red onion, pickles, and half the dill. In a small bowl, whisk together the oil, vinegar, mustard, salt, and pepper until blended. Pour the dressing over the vegetables, gently folding to combine.

Serve at room temperature or chilled. Just before serving, spoon the peas over the salad, lay the sardines on top, and sprinkle the remaining dill over it all.

Vegan version

Instead of sardines, use organic non-GMO dried tofu. You also have the option to drink an extra serving of protein powder with dinner instead.

Shrimp and Quinoa Salad

PREP TIME: 15 MINUTES
COOK TIME: 10 MINUTES
SERVES 4

Shrimp and quinoa are great foods on their own, but when you bring them together you get the best of both worlds plus a little extra. This fresh, light dinner salad is made even better with the addition of some greens and cherry tomatoes. It's quick, easy, and full of flavor—exactly what you want for your dinner, if you ask me.

FOR THE SHRIMP

- 1 tablespoon olive oil
- 1 pound large shrimp, cleaned and deveined
- 2 garlic cloves, crushed
- Juice of $1/2$ lime
- Salt and pepper
- Sriracha or other hot sauce, to taste (optional)
- 1 tablespoon chopped fresh cilantro

FOR THE SALAD

- 1 cup cooked quinoa, unseasoned
- 1 cup chopped fresh spinach
- $1/4$ cup chopped fresh parsley
- $1/4$ cup chopped fresh cilantro
- $1/4$ cup chopped green onions
- 1 (16-ounce) can chickpeas, drained and rinsed

FOR THE DRESSING

- Zest and juice of $1/2$ lemon
- 1 tablespoon tahini
- 2 tablespoons olive oil
- 1 to 2 garlic cloves, crushed
- Salt and pepper

MAKE THE SHRIMP Heat the oil in a skillet over medium-high heat. Add the shrimp, garlic, lime juice, salt, and pepper. Cook until half done, about 2 minutes, then add the hot sauce, if using. Continue to cook until the shrimp is pink and opaque, about 5 minutes. Top with the cilantro.

MAKE THE SALAD In a bowl, stir together the quinoa, spinach, parsley, cilantro, green onions, and chickpeas.

<u>**MAKE THE DRESSING**</u> In a small bowl, combine the lemon juice and zest, tahini, oil, garlic, and salt and pepper.

Pour the dressing over the quinoa mixture, add the shrimp, and serve.

Vegan version

Instead of the shrimp, feel free to use organic and non-GMO extra-firm tofu seasoned with 1 teaspoon of nutritional yeast. You also have the option to drink an extra serving of protein powder with dinner instead.

Leftovers

If you have any leftover salad, make a yummy salad jar. Layer in the salad and the shrimp and enjoy for dinner the next day.

HEARTIER MEALS

Shepherd's Pie

PREP TIME: 10 MINUTES
COOK TIME: 40 MINUTES
SERVES 4

This has to be one of my absolute favorite recipes. It really redefines what you think of as "comfort food." Instead of a topping of mashed potatoes, this uses mashed cauliflower. It's perfect for fall or winter, and tastes just as good heated up the next day. What's not to love about that?

- 1 tablespoon olive oil
- 1 or 2 garlic cloves, chopped
- 1 large shallot, sliced
- 1 large white onion, chopped
- 1½ pounds ground turkey
- ½ teaspoon dried thyme
- 2 cups sliced carrots
- ¼ cup sliced celery
- 1 large zucchini, cubed
- ¼ teaspoon salt
- 3 cups cooked and mashed cauliflower

Preheat the oven to 350°F.

Heat the oil in a skillet over medium heat. Add the garlic, shallot, and onion, and sauté until soft and translucent, about 3 minutes. Add the turkey, breaking it up with a spatula, then add the thyme, carrots, celery, zucchini, and salt. Continue to cook until the vegetables are tender most of the way; they don't have to be completely cooked because they will bake some more in the oven.

Transfer the turkey mixture to a 9 by 13-inch baking dish. Spread the mashed cauliflower over, dragging it with a fork, lightly, across the top to "rough up" the surface.

Bake the pie for 30 minutes, or until nicely browned on top and the filling is bubbling up a bit at the edges. Cut into 12 sections, and let cool a bit before serving.

Vegan version

Instead of the turkey, feel free to use organic non-GMO crumbled tempeh. You also have the option to drink an extra serving of protein powder with dinner instead.

Leftovers

Cover tightly and refrigerate any leftover sections. They make the perfect meal the next day, and they freeze exceptionally well.

Savory and Sweet Stuffed Cabbage

PREP TIME: 10 MINUTES
COOK TIME: 2 HOURS 10 MINUTES
SERVES 8

Have a little bit more time to dedicate to dinner? You won't be disappointed with this recipe. An equal combination of savory and sweet, the cabbage makes a great vehicle to carry a selection of other flavors—like organic raisins, for instance!

- 1 medium head of green cabbage
- Avocado oil cooking spray
- $\frac{1}{2}$ medium white onion, diced
- 3 garlic cloves, chopped
- $\frac{1}{4}$ cup sun-dried tomatoes (optional)
- 1 teaspoon dried basil

- 1 pound ground beef (ideally lean and grass-fed; see Tip)
- Smoked paprika
- Salt and pepper
- 6 large carrots, shredded
- $\frac{1}{4}$ cup (organic) raisins
- 1 (14.5-ounce) jar tomato sauce

Preheat the oven to 350°F.

You need to soften the cabbage, and you can do it in one of two ways: core the cabbage and then either microwave it cored side down for 7 minutes, or simmer it in boiling water until the leaves soften. Remove the leaves as they soften and dunk them in a bowl of ice water. Dry the leaves, continuing to soften until you have 8 good, whole leaves for stuffing.

Spray the oil on a skillet set over medium-high heat and then sauté the onion until translucent, about 3 minutes. Add the garlic, tomatoes if using, and the basil. Cook for 1 to 2 minutes, or until fragrant. Add the beef, breaking it up a bit with a spatula while mixing with the onion in the pan. Cook for 3 to 4 minutes, until just lightly browned. Add the paprika, salt, and pepper to taste; mix well.

Spread the cabbage leaves open on the counter and fill the centers of each with some of the meat mixture. Add the carrots and raisins, distributing them among the leaves. Roll up the cabbage leaves.

Spread some of the tomato sauce in a baking dish that will hold the 8 stuffed cabbages. Place the cabbage rolls on top of the sauce, then spread the remaining tomato sauce over the top and sprinkle on any remaining stuffing.

Cover the dish with foil and bake for 2 hours, or until the sauce is bubbly.

Tip

If you don't want to use grass-fed beef, substitute ground pork or lean ground turkey.

Vegan version

Instead of the ground meat, feel free to use organic non-GMO crumbled tempeh or pressed and crumbled extra-firm tofu. To make pressed tofu, slice the tofu into $1/2$-inch sections, lay on a towel, place a towel over the top, and add a weight like a heavy pan or cutting board. Let sit for 30 minutes. You also have the option to drink an extra serving of protein powder with dinner instead.

Leftovers

Cover the dish tightly and refrigerate the remainder for enjoying the next day, when it is even tastier.

Vegan Pumpkin Risotto

PREP TIME: 5 MINUTES

COOK TIME: 30 MINUTES

SERVES 6

I'm a big fan of vegan and vegetarian twists on classic recipes, and this pumpkin risotto is one of them! The pumpkin adds a sweet and unique flavor, which is perfect for fall as a vegetarian Thanksgiving entree or even an anytime dinner.

- 1 tablespoon olive oil
- 1 medium white onion, diced
- 2 cups arborio (or other short-grain) rice (see Tip)
- 1 cup cooking wine
- 4 cups vegetable broth, heated

- 1 cup canned pumpkin puree
- 1 teaspoon grated fresh ginger
- 1 teaspoon ground nutmeg
- 1 tablespoon chopped fresh basil
- Salt and pepper

Heat the oil in a large skillet over medium heat. Add the onion and sauté until soft and translucent, 3 to 5 minutes. Add the rice, and sauté, stirring, for 1 to 2 minutes. Slowly add the wine and stir, scraping up any browned particles. After the wine is absorbed by the rice, start adding the broth $1/2$ cup at a time. Let the rice absorb the broth before adding the next $1/2$ cup. Stir frequently and keep the risotto cooking at a gentle simmer until the broth is all absorbed and the rice kernels are swollen and tender but not yet mushy, about 20 minutes.

Stir in the pumpkin, ginger, nutmeg, and basil. Season to taste with salt and pepper. Heat just until everything is warmed throughout, then serve.

Tip

If you have a gluten allergy, be sure to use certified gluten-free arborio rice in order to avoid any cross-contamination.

Fall Vegetable Beef Roast

PREP TIME: 10 MINUTES
COOK TIME: 3 TO 4 HOURS
SERVES 6

Even though I live in the desert, when the weather starts to turn cold I always turn to this hearty beef recipe. It's a nice collection of vegetables that, through long and slow cooking, really get the time to soak up all the flavors. This dish just warms you up, inside and out.

- 1 tablespoon extra-virgin olive oil
- 1 teaspoon sea salt
- 1 teaspoon freshly ground black pepper
- 1 2- to 3-pound (organic) boneless beef chuck roast
- 2 teaspoons dried thyme
- 1 medium onion, cut into chunks
- 2 cups (organic) vegetable juice cocktail or tomato puree

- 2 cups (organic) beef broth
- 3 or 4 large carrots, cut into 3-inch pieces
- 4 or 5 red potatoes, cut into large chunks
- 1 rutabaga (yellow turnip) or sweet potato, peeled and cut into large chunks
- 3 celery stalks, cut into 3-inch pieces
- Sea salt or Herbamare

Preheat the oven to 325°F.

Heat the olive oil in a large Dutch oven set over medium-high heat. Rub the salt and pepper into the meat on all sides. Add the meat to the Dutch oven, and sear for a few minutes on each side. Add the thyme, onion, vegetable juice, and broth.

Cover, transfer to the oven, and braise for 2 hours, or until the meat is firm but starting to get tender.

Add the carrots, potatoes, rutabaga, and celery, then return the pot to the oven and cook for an additional 1 to 2 hours, or until the meat is so tender it begins to fall apart and the vegetables are cooked through. Let cool briefly, then season to taste with the salt and serve.

Vegan version

Instead of the beef, feel free to use organic non-GMO seasoned tempeh. You also have the option to drink an extra serving of protein powder with dinner instead.

Asparagus and Sweet Potato Skillet

PREP TIME: 5 MINUTES
COOK TIME: 25 MINUTES
SERVES 4

Skillet recipes are some of the easiest and most delicious meals you can prepare in a hurry. Packed with fiber, folate, chromium, vitamins A, C, E, and K, the asparagus combines with the sweet potato to make a delicious, healthy dinner that's perfect for sharing with friends who stop by.

- 1 pound boneless, skinless chicken breasts
- Sea salt and freshly ground black pepper
- 1 tablespoon olive oil
- 3 garlic cloves, minced
- 1 medium sweet potato, peeled and diced
- $1/2$ cup chicken broth or water
- $1/2$ pound fresh asparagus, stems trimmed and cut on diagonal into 2-inch lengths
- $1/2$ teaspoon red pepper flakes

Dice the chicken and season with salt and pepper.

Put the oil in a skillet set over medium heat. Add the garlic and then the chicken, and sauté, stirring, for 7 to 10 minutes, or until cooked through. Set the chicken aside.

To the same skillet, add the sweet potato and broth. Cook over medium heat until the sweet potato cubes are tender, 7 to 10 minutes.

Add the asparagus and cook for 4 to 5 minutes, or until fork-tender. Season to taste with salt and pepper, and sprinkle on the red pepper flakes. Serve at once.

Serving suggestions

This recipe becomes even heartier when served over a bed of tender brown rice.

Vegan version

Instead of the chicken, feel free to use Quorn meatless and soy-free chicken cutlets. Additionally, substitute vegetable broth for the chicken broth. You also have the option to drink an extra serving of protein powder with dinner instead.

Leftovers

Wrap any leftovers and refrigerate to enjoy in a wrap the next day.

Broccolini Chicken and Rice

PREP TIME: 5 MINUTES
COOK TIME: 35 MINUTES
SERVES 4

This is a super-simple dinner recipe that you're sure to enjoy time and time again. The best part? It also is a great leftover the next day. Feel free to add ¼ cup of nutritional yeast to this recipe, in order to add cheesy flavor.

- 2 tablespoons olive oil
- 1 cup cherry tomatoes
- 8 ounces (organic) chicken sausage (preferably seasoned only with salt and optionally onion or garlic), cut into small rounds
- 2 bunches broccolini, chopped
- Sea salt and freshly ground pepper
- 2 garlic cloves, minced
- 1 cup forbidden rice (also known as black rice) or wild rice
- 2½ cups chicken broth

Heat the oil in a large skillet (with a lid) over medium-high heat. Add the tomatoes and sauté for a few minutes. Add the sausage and brown evenly on both sides, about 5 minutes. Set aside.

Add the broccolini to the skillet. Season to taste with salt and pepper, and sauté until vibrant green and almost tender, about 5 minutes.

Add the garlic and rice, sautéing until fragrant, about 1 minute. Then add the sausage and the broth, and bring the mixture to a boil. Cover, reduce to a simmer, and cook until the liquid is absorbed and the rice is ready, about 30 minutes. Serve at once.

Vegan version

Instead of the chicken, feel free to use tempeh, tofu, or edamame, using organic and non-GMO products for the soy foods. Other options include spirulina or nutritional yeast. You also have the option to drink an extra serving of protein powder with dinner instead.

Leftovers

Make double the amount, then pack the leftovers in mason jars and use them for the next few days as delicious meals.

Creamy Basil and Chicken

PREP TIME: 5 MINUTES

COOK TIME: 35 MINUTES

SERVES 4

How much do you know about the potential value of basil for your life? Not only is it an adrenal adaptogen but it also provides polyphenols that protect your mitochondria. And it's delicious, making the perfect flavoring for this chicken dish.

- 1 teaspoon avocado oil
- $\frac{1}{2}$ cup chopped yellow onion
- 1 pound (organic) boneless, skinless chicken breasts, sliced into 4 cutlets
- 3 garlic cloves
- 2 tablespoons sunflower seeds
- 1 tablespoon nutritional yeast

- Salt and pepper
- 2 bunches fresh basil
- 1 tablespoon olive oil
- $\frac{1}{2}$ teaspoon arrowroot powder
- $\frac{1}{3}$ cup cold water
- $\frac{1}{2}$ cup coconut milk
- 1 cup cherry tomatoes, sliced in half

Heat the avocado oil in a large skillet over medium heat until it sizzles. Add the onion and cook for 3 to 4 minutes, until translucent. Add the chicken cutlets and cook for 12 minutes on one side, then flip and cook 13 minutes more on the other side, or until cooked through and the juices run clear when poked with a fork.

Meanwhile, prepare the pesto: Place the garlic in a food processor and pulse until finely minced. Add the sunflower seeds, and pulse several times more. Add the nutritional yeast, a sprinkle of salt, and a dash of pepper. Finally, add the basil and olive oil. Pulse until the basil is well minced and the mixture is blended.

In a small bowl, whisk the arrowroot powder into the cold water. Add the coconut milk, and then whisk in the pesto. Pour this sauce into the skillet around the chicken cutlets.

Briefly simmer the chicken and sauce in the pan until heated through. Add the cherry tomatoes, stir, and simmer for 1 to 2 more minutes, until the tomatoes are warmed. Serve at once.

Serving suggestions

This chicken dish can also be served over brown rice.

Vegan version

Instead of the chicken, feel free to use tempeh, tofu, or edamame, using organic and non-GMO products for the soy foods. Other options include spirulina or nutritional yeast. You also have the option to drink an extra serving of protein powder with dinner instead.

Unbeatable Minestrone

PREP TIME: 15 MINUTES
COOK TIME: 35 MINUTES
SERVES 8 TO 10

This hearty soup is not only great for you but also perfect for sharing with others. The recipe makes a lot, so there's lots to go around. It's full of flavor and has beautiful color—kids will love it, too. This is the perfect meal for those nights when you're craving delicious, good-for-you ingredients.

This recipe is thoroughly customizable; you could add other vegetables or protein. For example, try adding a cup of shredded chicken (or steamed white fish) to get more protein, more flavor, and more benefits from this delicious soup.

- 1$\frac{1}{2}$ cups (gluten-free) pasta
- 2 tablespoons olive oil
- 6 garlic cloves, chopped
- 1 (16-ounce) container cherry tomatoes
- 2 large carrots, chopped
- 3 celery stalks, chopped
- 1 large yellow onion, chopped
- 1 tablespoon chopped fresh thyme
- 1 (15-ounce) can red kidney beans, rinsed and drained
- 1 (15-ounce) can white kidney beans, rinsed and drained
- 1 (15-ounce) can chickpeas, rinsed and drained
- 1 (14.5-ounce) can diced tomatoes, with liquid
- 2 medium zucchini, chopped
- 8 cups (organic) chicken or vegetable broth
- 2 teaspoons black pepper
- 1 teaspoon salt

Cook the pasta according to package directions until al dente, then drain and toss with 1 tablespoon olive oil.

In a large pan or deep pot over medium heat, add the remaining tablespoon olive oil to warm for 30 seconds. Add the garlic, cherry tomatoes, carrots, celery, and onion. Cook until vegetables are soft, stirring often, about 10 minutes.

Add the thyme and raise the heat to high. Add the beans, chickpeas, diced tomatoes, and zucchini. Pour in the broth and bring to a boil. Lower the heat and simmer for 15 to 20 minutes, skimming off any foam that forms on the top.

Season with pepper and salt, then stir in the pasta. Heat through and then serve.

Vegan options

To make this recipe vegan, replace the chicken broth with vegetable broth.

Grilled Chicken with Blackberry Salsa

PREP TIME: 25 MINUTES (INCLUDES MARINATING)
COOK TIME: 10 MINUTES
SERVES 4

This tasty meal is a snap, especially when you're in a rush. This is the perfect summer dish—or even when you want a reminder of summer. The blackberry salsa is an especially exciting addition, as it lends a sweet element that is just too good to pass up.

- 2 tablespoons olive oil
- 1 teaspoon salt, plus more as needed
- 1 teaspoon ground cumin
- 2 limes
- 4 (organic) chicken breast, halves or cutlets
- 1 cup blackberries, coarsely chopped
- 1 cup (organic, non-GMO) cooked fresh or thawed frozen corn kernels
- 1 jalapeño, thinly sliced, seeds and ribs removed if desired
- 1 medium avocado
- Chopped fresh cilantro

Heat an outdoor grill, or grill pan on the stovetop, to high heat.

Place the oil, salt, and cumin in a large resealable bag. Finely grate the zest of 1 lime and add it to the bag. Juice the lime as well, adding the juice to the bag. Mix to combine, then add the chicken breasts, seal the bag, and refrigerate for 15 minutes.

Zest and juice the remaining lime and place the zest and juice in a small bowl. Add the blackberries, corn, and jalapeño. Dice the avocado and add to the bowl as well. Season with a pinch of salt and stir to combine.

When the grill is ready, remove the chicken from the marinade and place on the grill. Grill until the chicken is cooked through, 6 to 8 minutes per side. Remove from the grill, place on a cutting board, and let stand 5 minutes before slicing. Top the servings with the blackberry salsa and sprinkle each with a little cilantro.

Serving suggestion

To round out your good carbs and make this a truly dazzlingly colorful dish, serve alongside some steamed orange lentils.

Vegan version

Instead of the chicken, feel free to use Quorn meatless and soy-free chicken cutlets or organic and non-GMO firm tofu. You also have the option to drink an extra serving of protein powder with dinner instead.

Spicy Shrimp and Beans

PREP TIME: 25 MINUTES
COOK TIME: 10 MINUTES
SERVES 4

Can shrimp be good for you? The short answer is yes, if you're careful choosing the right type. Wild-caught shrimp are packed with nutrients, like tryptophan, B_{12}, selenium, astaxanthin, omega-3 fats, and even zinc. It's no wonder shrimp is good for brain aging and exceptional for bone health—which is why I share this recipe with you.

- 2 tablespoons olive oil
- 1 pound (wild-caught) shrimp, peeled and deveined
- $1/4$ teaspoon red pepper flakes
- 2 garlic cloves, minced
- $1/4$ cup apple cider vinegar
- 2 (15-ounce) cans white beans, drained and rinsed
- 1 pint cherry tomatoes, cut into halves
- Kosher salt
- $1/4$ cup coarsely chopped fresh parsley leaves
- 2 cups cooked long-grain jasmine brown rice, warmed

Heat the oil in a large skillet (with a lid) over medium-low heat. Add the shrimp and cook for 2 minutes. Set aside.

Add the red pepper flakes and garlic to the skillet and cook until fragrant, about 1 minute. Pour in the vinegar and simmer an additional minute. Mix in the beans and cherry tomatoes, then season the mixture with salt to taste.

Add the shrimp to the skillet and gently toss to combine. Cover and simmer until the shrimp are cooked through, about 3 to 5 minutes. Sprinkle with the parsley and serve over the rice.

Vegan version

Instead of the shrimp, feel free to use non-GMO extra-firm tofu. Crumble into bite-sized pieces and use in place of the shrimp. Add $1/2$ teaspoon of nutritional yeast at the end of the cooking to get some of the umami flavor. You also have the option to drink an extra serving of protein powder with dinner instead.

Leftovers

Double the quantity of shrimp and cook as directed, then wrap and refrigerate overnight to enjoy tomorrow as a light dinner.

Best Thai Chicken Coconut Soup

PREP TIME: 10 MINUTES
COOK TIME: 15 MINUTES
SERVES 4

There's just something about soup that makes me feel good, especially when it has just the right amount of spice. That's what this hearty Thai-style chicken coconut soup is all about, especially because it is so simple. All you need is a handful of ingredients and a slow cooker (optional) or Dutch oven, and you'll be enjoying this amazing dinner in no time—well, in 4 to 8 hours, actually! Substitute an Anaheim chile for the Thai, if you prefer it not quite as hot.

- 1 teaspoon grated lime zest
- $1/4$ cup fresh lime juice
- 1 tablespoon chopped lemongrass
- 2 tablespoons Thai fish sauce (Red Boat is good brand)
- $1/2$ teaspoon minced fresh ginger

- $1/2$ teaspoon minced seeded fresh Thai chile (optional)
- 1 pound (organic) chicken breast, cut into bite-sized pieces
- 1 (8.5-ounce) can light coconut milk
- 2 tablespoons chopped fresh cilantro

Combine the lime zest, lime juice, lemongrass, fish sauce, ginger, and chile in a large saucepan over medium heat. Bring to a simmer and then stir in the chicken and coconut milk. Cook for about 10 minutes, or until the chicken is cooked through and the flavors have blended. Sprinkle with the cilantro and serve immediately.

Tip

As an alternative, you can assemble these ingredients in a slow cooker and set on high for 4 hours or on low for 6 to 8 hours, to enjoy hours later.

Vegan version

Instead of the chicken, feel free to use Quorn meatless and soy-free chicken cutlets or organic and non-GMO tempeh cut into bite-sized pieces. Also, omit the fish sauce; nutritional yeast makes a good vegan substitute for that same umami flavor. You also have the option to drink an extra serving of protein powder with dinner instead.

Sesame Beef and Broccoli

PREP TIME: 20 MINUTES (INCLUDES 10 MINUTES REST TIME)
COOK TIME: 20 MINUTES
SERVES 6

This is a great recipe when you're looking for a simple combination of protein and vegetables. An under-the-radar addition here is the arrowroot flour. It's a nongrain, wheat-free flour that does a fantastic job of thickening sauces and makes a healthy breading for sautéed foods. It's also got resistant starch, is high in potassium, is alkalizing, slowly digests in the body, and is good for your gut flora. What's not to love about that? Let's get cooking!

- $1/3$ cup (wheat-free, organic, non-GMO) tamari
- $1/4$ cup arrowroot flour
- $1/4$ cup toasted sesame oil
- 3 garlic cloves, minced
- 1 2-inch piece fresh ginger, grated
- $2 1/2$ pounds (grass-fed) beef flank steak
- 4 cups broccoli florets
- 2 cups halved shiitake mushrooms
- 2 tablespoons extra-virgin olive oil

Preheat the oven to 375°F and line a large baking sheet with foil.

Whisk the tamari, arrowroot flour, sesame oil, garlic, and ginger together in a small bowl. Measure $1/4$ cup of the marinade and set aside. Rub the remaining marinade into the steak, coating both sides well.

Spread the broccoli florets and mushrooms on the baking sheet, drizzle with the olive oil, and add the marinade, turning to coat the vegetables. Roast until just tender, about 10 minutes. Remove the baking sheet from the oven and set the oven to broil.

Push the broccoli and mushrooms to the edges of the baking sheet, and place the steak in the center. Drizzle any remaining marinade over the steak, then slide the baking sheet under the broiler, and broil until the steak begins to char, 3 to 5 minutes. Turn over and broil the other side, another 3 minutes. This gives you a steak that is medium-rare; broil longer if you prefer better done.

Let the steak rest, loosely covered with foil, for 10 minutes to set the juices. Then slice the steak across the grain and serve along with the roasted broccoli and mushrooms.

Serving suggestions

The steak and veggies can be also served over or with brown rice or quinoa.

Vegan version

Instead of the beef, feel free to use thinly sliced organic and non-GMO tempeh or tofu. For best flavor, marinate for 20 minutes before broiling. You also have the option to drink an extra serving of protein powder with dinner instead.

Easy Slow Cooker Chicken

PREP TIME: 5 MINUTES
COOK TIME: 4 HOURS
SERVES 4
SPECIAL EQUIPMENT: SLOW COOKER

This is a simple dinner you can always rely on—all you need is an onion, a chicken, a slow cooker, and 4 hours!

- 1 large onion, sliced
- 1 3-pound chicken

Lay the onion slices in the bottom of a slow cooker. Place the whole chicken, breast side down, on top. Cover and cook on high for 4 hours.

Serving suggestions

Pair this slow-cooked chicken with a simple green salad.

Leftovers

Pair any remaining chicken with cooked brown rice or quinoa for dinner the next day.

Baked Shrimp with Lemon and Chives

PREP TIME: 10 MINUTES
COOK TIME: 15 MINUTES
SERVES 4

What are the elements of a truly perfect meal? It has to be easy, with only a few ingredients; it needs to be fast (especially if you're in a rush for dinner); and it has to be healthy and delicious. These shrimp are all that and more! Don't blame me if you end up wanting these every night for dinner.

- 2 pounds (wild-caught) shrimp, peeled and deveined
- Juice of 1 lemon
- 1 teaspoon salt
- Freshly ground black pepper
- 1 tablespoon fresh or freeze-dried chopped chives

Preheat the oven to 425°F. Line a baking sheet with unbleached parchment.

Spread the shrimp on the baking sheet, making sure they don't overlap. Sprinkle the lemon juice over and season with salt and pepper. Bake for about 15 minutes, or until the shrimp turn pink. Add the chives and serve.

Serving suggestions

Pair this shrimp recipe with greens and carbs.

Vegan version

Instead of the shrimp, feel free to use frozen organic and non-GMO edamame. You also have the option to drink an extra serving of protein powder with dinner instead.

Zucchini Noodles with Baked Shrimp and Tomatoes

PREP TIME: 15 MINUTES (INCLUDES TIME FOR SPIRALIZING)
COOK TIME: 15 MINUTES
SERVES 4
SPECIAL EQUIPMENT: SPIRALIZER

When it comes to dinner at our house, the more vegetables, the better! This recipe relies on fresh noodles made from zucchini, which can be cooked to have that perfect crunch or to the point where they are nicely soft—it's entirely your choice. The shrimp add some quality protein, and the cherry tomatoes provide that pop of color.

- 2 pounds (wild-caught) shrimp, peeled and deveined
- 4 tablespoons avocado oil
- Juice of $\frac{1}{2}$ lemon
- $\frac{1}{2}$ medium yellow onion, chopped
- 3 garlic cloves, minced
- 1 pound cherry tomatoes, cut in halves
- $\frac{1}{4}$ cup finely chopped fresh basil
- 2 medium zucchini, spiralized
- Salt and pepper

Preheat the oven to 425°F. Line a baking sheet with unbleached parchment.

Spread the shrimp on the baking sheet, making sure they don't overlap. Season with about 2 tablespoons oil and the lemon juice. Bake for 15 minutes, or until the shrimp have turned pink.

Meanwhile, heat the remaining 2 tablespoons oil in a skillet over medium-high heat. Add the onion and sauté until slightly translucent, about 2 minutes. Add the garlic, tomatoes, and basil. Sauté and stir, occasionally, for 10 minutes.

Add the zucchini noodles to the skillet, and stir occasionally until cooked to your preferred consistency, from al dente to soft. Add salt and pepper to taste.

Serving suggestions

Feel free to enjoy this recipe with a separate side of carbs.

Vegan version

Instead of the shrimp, feel free to use tempeh, tofu, or edamame, using organic and non-GMO products for the soy foods. Other options include spirulina or nutritional yeast. You also have the option to drink an extra serving of protein powder with dinner instead.

Leftovers

Zucchini noodles are best enjoyed fresh, but if you have extra shrimp, you can wrap and refrigerate them to have the next day, perhaps with a new batch of spiralized zucchini noodles.

Sweet Potato Turkey Casserole

PREP TIME: 10 MINUTES

COOK TIME: 1 HOUR 10 MINUTES

SERVES 4-6

SPECIAL EQUIPMENT: SPIRALIZER

This dish is the perfect comfort food, yet it makes for a great dinner that's not too heavy. Also, it's a wonderful way to get good protein and other nutrients into your life. The best of all? It's perfect for sharing, and even more perfect for leftovers!

- $1\frac{1}{2}$ tablespoons extra-virgin olive oil, plus more for brushing
- 1 pound extra-lean (organic) ground turkey
- 1 tablespoon minced garlic
- $\frac{1}{4}$ cup chopped onion
- 1 (8-ounce) can tomato paste
- 1 (15-ounce) can petite diced tomatoes, drained
- 1 medium sweet potato, peeled and spiralized
- 1 medium zucchini, sliced into $\frac{1}{2}$-inch pieces

- $\frac{1}{2}$ teaspoon sea salt
- $\frac{1}{2}$ teaspoon black pepper
- $\frac{1}{4}$ teaspoon chili powder
- $\frac{1}{4}$ teaspoon ground cumin
- $\frac{1}{8}$ teaspoon dried oregano
- $\frac{1}{8}$ teaspoon ground cardamom
- 1 tablespoon almond flour
- 1 tablespoon coconut flour
- 1 cup unsweetened flax milk (or vegetable broth)

Preheat the oven to 350°F. Lightly brush a casserole dish with some oil.

Heat a large skillet over medium heat and add the turkey, garlic, and onion. Cook until lightly browned, about 5 minutes. Use a spatula to break up the meat as it browns. Stir in the tomato paste and tomatoes, and combine with the turkey. Add the sweet potato, cooking until slightly softened, about 3 minutes.

Place the zucchini in a bowl and mix in the salt, pepper, chili powder, cumin, oregano, and cardamom. Spread the zucchini mixture on the bottom of the casserole dish. Top with the turkey and sweet potato mixture. Place the casserole dish in the oven, and bake for 15 minutes.

Heat a small pot over high heat and add the olive oil along with both the almond and coconut flours. Stir for 1 minute, until thickened. Reduce to medium-high heat and slowly add the flax milk, whisking and simmering the sauce for another 2 minutes.

Remove the casserole from the oven and pour in the sauce. Continue to bake for another 40 to 45 minutes, until the top of the casserole has lightly browned. Let cool slightly, then slice this casserole into 4 to 6 equal pieces and serve immediately.

Vegan version

Instead of the turkey, feel free to use organic and non-GMO tempeh or extra-firm tofu. You also have the option to drink an extra serving of protein powder with dinner instead.

Leftovers

Comfort foods just have a way of tasting even better the next day. If you have leftovers, cover them tightly and refrigerate to enjoy again tomorrow.

Wild Salmon with Ginger-Lime Marinade

PREP TIME: 45 MINUTES TO 2½ HOURS (INCLUDES MARINATING TIME)

COOK TIME: 25 MINUTES

SERVES 4

What's not to love about salmon? It pairs delightfully with this great ginger-lime marinade. In fact, the distinct flavor of the ginger, paired with the acidity of the lime, really bring out extra flavor from the salmon—it might just have you jumping (upstream) for joy!

- 1 pound (wild-caught) Alaskan salmon fillet
- ½ cup tamari
- Juice of 1 lime
- 1 teaspoon grated fresh ginger
- 2 to 4 garlic cloves, crushed
- Few dashes of hot pepper sesame oil

Place the salmon skin side up in a glass baking dish. Mix the tamari, lime juice, ginger, garlic to taste, and hot oil in a small bowl, then pour over the salmon. Cover the dish and marinate in the refrigerator for 30 minutes to 2 hours.

When ready to bake, preheat the oven to 400°F. Drain the marinade off the salmon, and flip the salmon skin side down. Transfer the baking dish to the oven and bake for 15 to 25 minutes, depending on the thickness of the fillet (figure 10 minutes per 1 inch of thickness). Serve.

Serving suggestions

This salmon pairs perfectly with a fresh side of greens.

Vegan version

Instead of the salmon, feel free to use tempeh, tofu, or edamame, using organic and non-GMO products for the soy foods. Other options include spirulina or nutritional yeast. You also have the option to drink an extra serving of protein powder with dinner instead.

SALADS

Seared Cod with Chilled Potatoes

PREP TIME: 30 MINUTES (INCLUDES COOKING THE VEGETABLES)
COOK TIME: 10 MINUTES
SERVES 4

How do you enjoy potatoes while preserving all that good resistant starch? That's easy—you serve them chilled! Boiling preserves much of that starch, and when the boiled potatoes are refrigerated, they form even more starch in a process called "retrograde resistant starch formation." Paired with some delicious fish, this is a great meal to start or finish the week.

- 1 teaspoon macadamia nut oil or grapeseed oil
- 1 pound (wild-caught) Atlantic cod fillet
- 1 pound baby potatoes, boiled 20 minutes, then refrigerated overnight
- 1 pound green beans, boiled 10 minutes, then refrigerated overnight
- 1/4 cup diced red onion
- 1 tablespoon (soy-free vegan) mayonnaise

Heat the oil in a large sauté pan over medium-high heat, then sauté the cod on both sides, 6 to 8 minutes total, turning once, until flaky. Let cool slightly, then cut it into small pieces.

Dice the potatoes and beans, and mix with the onion in a large salad bowl. Add the mayonnaise, toss gently, and sprinkle the cod pieces on top.

Vegan version

Instead of the cod, feel free to add a serving of organic and non-GMO edamame as a side dish. You also have the option to drink an extra serving of protein powder with dinner instead.

Tomato, Cucumber, and Green Bean Salad with Walnut Dressing

PREP TIME: 75 MINUTES
COOK TIME: 6 MINUTES
SERVES 4

This salad chockful of veggies is sure to be a hit—as well as good for your health! For example, the green beans are high in resistant starch, and the vinegar slows your absorption of glucose. The fish sauce lends that umami that makes this combo unforgettable. And if you want to add protein to this meal, consider the addition of smoked tofu. It will give a smoky-spicy complexion to the salad for a different effect.

- 8 ounces (organic) green beans, trimmed and cut into 1-inch pieces
- $1/3$ cup walnut pieces
- 1 garlic clove, chopped
- 1 teaspoon coarse sea salt
- 3 tablespoons macadamia nut oil
- 3 tablespoons apple cider vinegar
- 1 pint (organic) grape tomatoes, cut in half
- $1/2$ cup thinly sliced red onion
- $1/2$ medium cucumber, peeled, halved lengthwise, seeded, and sliced
- $1/4$ cup coarsely chopped fresh cilantro
- $1/4$ cup coarsely chopped fresh dill
- $1/4$ cup coarsely chopped fresh mint
- $1/2$ teaspoon Thai fish sauce (Red Boat is a good brand)

Cook the beans in boiling salted water until crisp-tender, 4 to 6 minutes. Drain well, rinse with cold water, and spread on a clean kitchen towel to pat dry. Let cool for 1 hour.

Combine the walnuts, garlic, and salt in a food processor or blender and process until finely ground. Pour into a salad bowl and add the oil and vinegar, whisking until well blended.

Add the beans, the tomatoes, onion slices, cucumber, cilantro, dill, and mint, then sprinkle on the fish sauce and toss to blend. Serve at once.

Vegan option

To make this recipe vegan, omit the fish sauce.

Egg-Free Niçoise Salad

PREP TIME: 10 MINUTES
COOK TIME: 10 MINUTES
SERVES 4

When it comes to potlucks and parties, this is one of my all-time favorite recipes to bring to friends. It's not only that, but it's also a full meal that helps you stay on track. You can customize it by varying the healthy ingredients that make up this fantastic salad.

- 3 cups cubed Yukon Gold potatoes
- 2 tablespoons extra-virgin olive oil
- 2 tablespoons balsamic vinegar
- Salt and freshly ground pepper
- 4 cups torn butter lettuce, washed well

- 1 bell pepper, cored and sliced
- 1 medium red onion, sliced
- 1 medium cucumber, peeled and sliced
- 2 cups shredded cooked chicken
- 2 teaspoons dried chives

Bring a saucepan of water to a strong, rolling boil. Add the potatoes and cook for 8 to 10 minutes, or until firm but done. Drain and put into the fridge to cool.

In a large salad bowl, whisk together the olive oil, vinegar, and salt and pepper to taste. Add the lettuce on one side of the bowl, then put the bell pepper, red onion, and cucumber each in a small section of the bowl. Toss with the dressing, then add the chicken and chives. Toss again lightly and serve.

Vegan version

Instead of the chicken, feel free to use Quorn meatless and soy-free chicken cutlets. You also have the option to drink an extra serving of protein powder with dinner instead.

Potato and Salmon Salad

PREP TIME: 15 MINUTES (INCLUDES PREPPING THE OPTIONALS)
COOK TIME: 20 MINUTES
SERVES 4

Want to know the great thing about cooked red potatoes? They're packed with resistant fiber, which is super for your adrenals. Wild-caught salmon can be enjoyed as much as a few times a week, so this recipe is a great way to incorporate both—in this case, with canned salmon! Enjoy it for dinner one evening and then again the next day, it's so versatile. And don't forget about the toppings. They are a great way to get even more variety into your diet, which is what this recipe is all about.

- 1 pound small red potatoes, quartered
- 2 1/2 tablespoons red wine vinegar
- 1 teaspoon Dijon mustard
- Sea salt and freshly ground black pepper
- 1/4 cup (organic) olive oil

- 1 pound whole green beans, trimmed
- 2 (5-ounce) cans wild-caught salmon, packed in water, drained
- 1 small red onion, diced
- 2 tablespoons chopped fresh parsley
- Lettuce, for serving

OPTIONAL TOPPINGS

- 1 medium avocado, cut into bite-sized pieces
- 2 medium beets, cut into bite-sized pieces and boiled for 10 minutes

- 8 ounces Brussels sprouts, stems and outer leaves removed, cut into half, and boiled for 8 minutes

Bring a pot of salted water to a boil. Add the potatoes and cook for 5 to 10 minutes, until fork-tender. Remove with a slotted spoon, and place the potatoes in a large salad bowl. Save the water.

While the potatoes cook, prepare the vinaigrette: Whisk together the vinegar, mustard, salt, and pepper in a small bowl. Slowly add the olive oil while continuing to whisk until the vinaigrette emulsifies. Set aside.

Bring the potato water back to a boil. Add the green beans and cook about 4 minutes, until crisp-tender. Drain and pat dry.

Add the beans to the potatoes, along with the salmon, red onion, and parsley. Season with salt and pepper to taste. Add the vinaigrette and any additional toppings, then toss and serve over your choice of lettuce.

Vegan version

Instead of the salmon, feel free to use Quorn meatless and soy-free chicken cutlets or organic and non-GMO dried tofu cut into bite-sized pieces. You also have the option to drink an extra serving of protein powder with dinner instead.

Leftovers

Feel free to make a batch of quinoa, and pair it with any salad leftovers (sans lettuce) for tomorrow.

Chinese Quinoa Chicken Salad

PREP TIME: 20 MINUTES
COOK TIME: 5 MINUTES
SERVES 4

Depending on your mood, a good chicken salad can make all the difference when it comes time to make dinner. This salad is also perfect for those with any allergies, as it is simple, filling, and fully customizable. Who said salad can't be fun?

FOR THE SALAD

- 3 cups cooked quinoa
- 2 cups shredded cooked chicken breast
- $1/2$ cup shredded carrot
- $1/2$ cup minced red bell pepper
- 1 cup chopped fresh spinach
- 2 green onions, chopped
- $1/4$ cup peanuts, chopped
- $1/2$ cup finely chopped broccoli

FOR THE DRESSING

- 1 tablespoon cream-style (organic) peanut butter (or Sunbutter sunflower butter)
- 2 teaspoons toasted sesame oil
- 1 teaspoon (organic, non-GMO, gluten-free) tamari
- 1 teaspoon rice vinegar
- Juice of $1/2$ lime
- 2 to 3 tablespoons water

Combine all the salad ingredients except the broccoli in a large bowl.

Gently steam the broccoli for 2 minutes (or 40 seconds in a microwave on high), and transfer to the salad bowl. Toss to combine.

Combine the ingredients for the dressing and drizzle over the salad, tossing again so everything is incorporated and seasoned with dressing. Serve immediately or store in the fridge until serving time.

Vegan version

Instead of the chicken, feel free to use Quorn meatless and soy-free chicken nuggets or organic and non-GMO dried tofu cut into bite-sized pieces. You also have the option to drink an extra serving of protein powder with dinner instead.

UNLIMITED RECIPES

Carrot Fries

PREP TIME: 5 MINUTES
COOK TIME: 30 MINUTES
YIELD: VARIES

You might love french fries made with potatoes, but did you know that you can make fries out of carrots? Using this "unlimited" food, which makes them totally guilt-free, is a great alternative to the standard choice. Baked, not fried, and slightly charred so that you get that caramelized flavor, carrot fries are a great opportunity to try something different when it comes to snacking. Bear in mind that for some ovens, it may take a little longer to cook the carrots—as much as an additional 5 minutes on each side.

- Avocado oil cooking spray
- Carrots
- Salt

OPTIONAL SEASONINGS

- Smoked paprika
- Garlic powder
- Powdered rosemary
- Minced dried chives

Preheat the oven to 425°F. Lightly spray a baking sheet with cooking spray.

Cut your desired amount of carrots into small "fries." You can do this in one of the following ways: (1) using a knife, cut baby carrots into quarters lengthwise or cut standard carrots in half and then quarter them, or (2) use a veggie chopping tool that cuts foods into "fry-form."

Place the carrots on the baking sheet, trying not to let them touch. Lightly spray the carrots with the oil, then sprinkle with salt.

Bake for 15 minutes. Turn the fries over, or stir them around, and bake for another 15 minutes. The goal is for them to turn golden, or slightly charred, so they acquire a caramelized flavor.

When the carrots are done, add the optional seasonings. They are best served warm, right after roasting.

Beet "Chips"

PREP TIME: 5 MINUTES
COOK TIME: 20 MINUTES
MAKES 4 CUPS

These are honestly nothing like your everyday, run-of-the-mill chips. They are the perfect healthy snack and are easy to make. Beets contain an amino acid that fights heart disease, regulates hormones, and helps with detoxification. Having a mandolin is helpful here, but not essential. In terms of health, the appropriate number of beets to eat is $1/2$ cup in a cooked or juiced form two or three times a week; this is a fun way to make your beet quota.

- 3 medium to large beets, rinsed and scrubbed
- Avocado oil cooking spray
- Sea salt
- Freshly ground black pepper
- 2 or 3 rosemary sprigs, leaves roughly chopped

Preheat the oven to 375°F. Place the oven rack in the center of the oven. Line 2 baking sheets with parchment.

Thinly slice the beets with a mandolin or a sharp knife, getting them as consistently thin as possible. A good tip to know whether you're cutting them right is if they curl just a bit when cut; this helps ensure even baking and crispiness.

Divide the sliced beets between the baking sheets and spray with the cooking spray. Add a pinch of salt and pepper, and sprinkle on the rosemary. Toss to coat well.

Arrange the beets in a single layer, ensuring that the slices aren't touching. Bake for 15 to 20 minutes, or until crisp and slightly brown. Watch closely, as they can burn quickly. Remove, let cool slightly, and enjoy.

Chili-Roasted Carrots

PREP TIME: 5 MINUTES

COOK TIME: 25 MINUTES

MAKES 6 CUPS, OR 4 SERVINGS AS A SIDE DISH

Apart from bursting with flavor, these carrots are rich in vitamin A, which is exactly what your brain needs when it's craving an energy boost. These are a super snack but also make a great side dish for grilled chicken or pork.

- 1 tablespoon grapeseed oil
- 1 teaspoon chili powder
- 1 teaspoon ground cumin
- $\frac{1}{2}$ teaspoon sea salt
- 2 pounds carrots, cut into $\frac{1}{4}$-inch diagonal slices
- 2 tablespoons chopped fresh cilantro
- 2 tablespoons lime juice

Position a rack in the lower third of the oven. Preheat the oven to 450°F. Line a baking sheet with parchment.

Combine the oil, chili powder, cumin, and salt in a large bowl. Add the sliced carrots and toss well to coat. Spread the carrots on the baking sheet, then roast, stirring once, until tender and golden, 20 to 25 minutes.

Toss the roasted carrots with the cilantro and lime juice. Serve immediately.

Zesty Cucumber-Pepper Rainbow Salad

PREP TIME: 5 MINUTES
COOK TIME: 10 MINUTES
SERVES 4

Tired of salads with lettuce, and longing for something with zest and flavor? You have to try this. Chickpeas, as your good carb, olive oil and avocado for good fats, and a side of protein (chicken, for example) come together for this healthy twist on traditional salads. Feel free to add about 1 cup of shredded chicken, for additional protein.

- 3 medium cucumbers, peeled, seeded, and chopped
- 2 bell peppers of different colors, cored, seeded, and chopped
- 1 large ripe tomato, or $1/2$ pint cherry tomatoes
- $1/2$ medium avocado, cut into chunks
- $1/4$ medium onion (optional)
- 1 (15-ounce) can chickpeas, rinsed and drained
- Finely chopped fresh cilantro (optional)
- Juice of 1 lemon, or $1 1/2$ limes
- 2 tablespoons olive oil
- Sea salt and freshly ground pepper

In a large mixing bowl, combine the cucumbers, bell peppers, tomato, avocado, onion, and chickpeas. Sprinkle on the cilantro, if using, and the lemon juice and olive oil. Mix well, and season to taste with salt and pepper.

Leftovers

Because this salad has no lettuce, it keeps well in the fridge overnight.

Roasted Orange Pepper Soup

PREP TIME: 10 MINUTES
COOK TIME: 25 MINUTES
SERVES 4

This recipe relies on the subtle but delicious flavor of orange bell peppers. Not only do they lend the soup a generous thickness but they also provide a mild spiciness that I just love. It's an easy way to enjoy a delicious soup with our helpful "unlimited" foods. This soup has a medium rating for spiciness; if you like it mild, add only $1/2$ teaspoon red pepper flakes. An immersion blender is helpful here, although you could transfer the soup to a food processor or blender to puree.

- 1 tablespoon avocado oil
- 1 large sweet onion, diced
- 2 tablespoons chopped garlic
- $1/2$ to 1 teaspoon red pepper flakes
- 1 teaspoon sea salt (or Herbamare)
- 4 cups (organic) vegetable or chicken stock
- 4 to 5 orange bell peppers, roasted
- 4 cups chopped tomatoes
- $1/4$ cup minced fresh parsley
- $1/4$ cup minced fresh basil

Heat the oil in a 6-quart pot over medium heat. Add the onion, garlic, red pepper flakes, and salt. Sauté until the onion is translucent, about 3 minutes.

Add the stock, bell peppers, and tomatoes; lower the heat, cover, and simmer the mixture for 20 minutes, stirring occasionally.

Puree the soup in the pot using an immersion blender, or puree in batches in a food processor or blender, then return to the pot. Simmer the puree for 5 minutes, then add the parsley and basil, stir, and simmer for 5 additional minutes. Taste and adjust the seasonings if needed.

Leftovers

This soup holds well overnight, tightly covered and refrigerated, to be enjoyed the next day, whether as a lunch or a dinner.

Fresh Spring Gazpacho

PREP TIME: 3 TO 12 HOURS (INCLUDES OVERNIGHT CHILLING)
SERVES 4

This no-cook soup is absolutely perfect for spring or summer. Gazpacho is traditionally served cold, meaning it is refreshing when the days grow warmer. It's also a way for some of our favorite fresh herbs to steal the show. It's helpful to have an immersion blender, but a food processor also works well to puree the soup.

- 3 Roma (plum) tomatoes, peeled, seeded, and chopped (about 3 cups)

- 1 large cucumber, peeled, seeded, and chopped (about 2 cups)

- 1 red bell pepper, seeds and white ribs removed and chopped

- 1 medium white onion, chopped

- 3 cups canned tomato juice

- 2 tablespoons chopped fresh herbs (tarragon, thyme, parsley)

- ¼ cup red wine vinegar

- 2 garlic cloves, finely chopped

- 2 tablespoons tomato paste

- Juice of ½ lemon

- Sea salt

- Dash of cayenne pepper

Set aside 2 tablespoons each of the tomatoes, cucumber, bell pepper, and onion. Place the remaining in a large bowl. Add the tomato juice, herbs, vinegar, garlic, and tomato paste. Use an immersion blender to puree. Alternatively, place the ingredients in a food processor and process until smooth. If the mixture is too thick, add a little water to reach the desired consistency.

Taste and adjust the seasoning, adding the lemon juice, salt, and cayenne. Cover and chill thoroughly, at least 3 hours and preferably overnight. When ready to serve, ladle into individual bowls and garnish with the reserved fresh vegetables.

Beet and Fennel Soup

PREP TIME: 5 MINUTES
COOK TIME: 40 MINUTES
SERVES 4

How much do you know about fennel? This vegetable surely has an interesting taste, with notes of licorice that pair perfectly with the earthy taste of beets. When you bring them together, they really make a great soup. This is one of my favorite recipes, and I can't wait to share it with you, to add some hearty goodness to your next dinner.

- Olive oil
- 4 medium red beets (about 1 pound), peeled and diced
- $\frac{1}{4}$ cup water
- $\frac{1}{2}$ teaspoon ground cinnamon
- $\frac{1}{2}$ teaspoon chili powder
- 4 cups (organic) chicken broth

- $1\frac{3}{4}$ cups chopped fennel bulb, fronds chopped for garnish
- 1 tablespoon mild (organic) honey
- $\frac{1}{2}$ teaspoon sea salt
- $\frac{1}{3}$ teaspoon freshly ground white pepper

Pour a little olive oil into a large saucepan set over medium-high heat. Add the beets, water, cinnamon, and chili powder, and sauté until the beets are soft, about 5 minutes.

Add the broth, chopped fennel, and honey. Bring the mixture to a boil, reduce the heat, and simmer for 40 minutes, or until everything is tender.

Let the soup cool a bit, then pour into a blender (in batches) and puree or use an immersion blender to puree right in the pot. Add the salt and pepper, and pour into serving bowls. Garnish the bowls with some chopped fennel fronds.

Vegan options

To make this recipe vegan, substitute vegetable broth for the chicken broth and omit the honey.

Leftovers

The soup freezes well, or cover and refrigerate the soup for a great meal the next day.

Savory Eggplant Boats

PREP TIME: 25 MINUTES
COOK TIME: 20 MINUTES
SERVES 4

This baked eggplant dish is perfect for company but also is family fare. The servings are pre-portioned, in that each slice provides a tasty blend of eggplant and sauce. Warning: like apples, eggplants brown soon after you slice them, so wait to cut them just before cooking. Also, you'll need a grill pan for this recipe.

- Avocado oil cooking spray
- 1 medium yellow onion, chopped
- 2 red, yellow, or orange bell peppers, cored, seeded, and cut into long, wide sections
- 3 garlic cloves, minced
- 1 (8-ounce) bag baby spinach
- 2 medium eggplants, cut into $\frac{1}{2}$-inch sections (long thin eggplants work best)

- $\frac{1}{2}$ cup balsamic vinegar
- 2 tablespoons drained capers
- 2 pints cherry or grape tomatoes, cut into quarters, or 3 large ripe tomatoes, cut into $\frac{1}{2}$-inch chunks
- Dash of paprika
- Sea salt

Preheat the oven to 425°F. Line a baking sheet with parchment.

Heat a skillet over medium-high heat and lightly coat with avocado oil spray. Add the onion and sauté until translucent, 2 to 3 minutes. Add the bell peppers and sauté until softened, about 15 minutes, stirring frequently. If they get too dry, add a little water to keep them from sticking to the pan. Add the garlic and spinach to the pan, sauté for 2 to 3 minutes, then set aside.

Lightly spray the eggplant slices with avocado oil and, using a stovetop grill pan, grill the slices quickly on each side, turning once, 10 to 15 minutes total. As the slices are finished, transfer them to the baking sheet. When all the eggplant slices are on the baking sheet, spread them with the pepper mixture. Bake for 20 minutes, until the eggplant is soft.

Bring the vinegar to a boil in a medium saucepan and simmer until reduced by half.

Add the capers, then the tomatoes, and cook over high heat for 3 to 5 minutes; a thick sauce should form.

Top the roasted eggplant with the balsamic tomato sauce, then sprinkle with paprika and a pinch of salt. Serve warm.

Asian Broth

PREP TIME: 5 MINUTES
COOK TIME: 2 TO 3 HOURS
SERVES 4

Looking for a good broth or soup stock? Why not make your own! This Asian broth relies on delicious shiitake mushrooms to form the base, alongside some lemongrass and red pepper flakes. It's a great recipe that is fine enjoyed plain or can serve as the foundation for plenty of dishes.

- 6 cups (organic) chicken or vegetable broth
- 6 cups water
- 2 medium onions, skins left on, cut into chunks
- 1 head of garlic, cut in half
- 1 2-inch piece fresh ginger, sliced

- 3 celery stalks, chopped
- 3 medium carrots, chopped
- 3 to 4 cups chopped shiitake mushrooms
- 1 lemongrass stalk, chopped
- 1 teaspoon red pepper flakes
- 1 to 2 teaspoons sea salt

Place all the ingredients in an 8-quart stockpot. Bring to a boil, cover, and reduce the heat to low. Simmer for 2 to 3 hours.

Strain the broth into a large bowl. Serve immediately or cover and refrigerate for up to 7 days or freeze for longer periods.

Zucchini Noodles with Bruschetta

PREP TIME: 25 MINUTES (INCLUDES MARINATING TIME AND SPIRALIZING)
COOK TIME: 5 MINUTES
SERVES 4

There are so many beautiful foods you can make with a spiralizer, and these vegetable noodles are among the best. This "pasta" nicely substitutes for traditional noodles and repackages zucchini in a fun form that your whole family is sure to love. For a full meal, add a lean protein (like grilled chicken) to this dish.

- 2 Roma (plum) tomatoes, diced
- $1/4$ medium yellow onion, diced
- 3 to 5 tablespoons balsamic vinegar
- $1/4$ cup olive oil
- $1/4$ teaspoon finely chopped fresh basil
- 3 medium green zucchini
- Sea salt and freshly ground pepper

Mix the tomatoes, onion, vinegar, oil, and basil in a bowl and let marinate in the refrigerator for 15 minutes, stirring occasionally.

Meanwhile, use a spiralizer to make the zucchini noodles.

Heat a large skillet over medium-high heat. Add the zucchini noodles and gently cook for 5 minutes, keeping them still firm. Top with the marinated tomato mixture. Season to taste with salt and pepper. Spoon out the noodles and serve immediately.

Green Beans with Miso-Sesame Sauce

PREP TIME: 5 MINUTES
COOK TIME: 10 MINUTES
SERVES 4

Think of this recipe as an alternative to that traditional green bean casserole. The beans themselves are rich in chlorophyll, just like leafy greens, and are high in natural silicates, which make your hair and skin healthier. They also are a great source of fiber. So, what are you waiting for? Paired with miso, which is a super fermented food in and of itself, this dish makes a great side to just about any meal. And it is perfect as an anytime snack whenever you're hungry.

- 2 $\frac{1}{2}$ tablespoons white sesame seeds
- $\frac{1}{4}$ cup unseasoned Japanese rice vinegar
- 2 tablespoons (organic, naturally fermented, non-GMO) white miso paste
- 1 pound thin green beans, trimmed
- 1 teaspoon sea salt

Grind 2 tablespoons of the sesame seeds in a spice grinder, or put them in a plastic bag and mash with a rolling pin until they are a powder.

Combine the sesame seed powder with the vinegar and miso in a small bowl, and whisk until well blended. Set the sauce aside.

Fill a large saucepan three-fourths with water and bring to a boil. Add the beans and salt, and cook until tender to the bite, 6 to 8 minutes.

Drain the beans and place in a shallow serving bowl. Spoon the sauce over, and garnish with the remaining sesame seeds (and enjoy the added benefits of copper and phytosterols from the seeds).

Sautéed Greens with Lemon

PREP TIME: 5 MINUTES
COOK TIME: 5 MINUTES
SERVES 4

When was the last time you had mustard greens? They are perfect for making a large batch, as they keep well for up to three days when refrigerated. Beyond that, though, they offer a subtle kick—just like mustard—and are delicious when served warm. Toss them with your favorite dressing to enjoy as a quick meal. Best of all, they are cruciferous, which means you're also reducing your cancer risk and are safeguarding your thyroid. Now, that's a win-win-win situation.

- 2 bunches mustard greens, trimmed of stems
- 2 tablespoons macadamia nut oil
- $\frac{1}{4}$ teaspoon sea salt
- $\frac{1}{4}$ teaspoon black pepper
- Pinch of cayenne pepper

Toss the greens in a bowl with 1 tablespoon of the oil and the salt, black pepper, and cayenne pepper.

Heat the remaining tablespoon oil in a large skillet over high heat. Add the greens, in batches, stirring frequently, and cook until wilted, about 2 minutes. Serve warm.

Leftovers

Cooked mustard greens keep well, covered, in the refrigerator for up to 3 days.

chapter nine

Maintenance

Now that you have improved your liver function, your metabolism will work better. You have the chance to start a whole new chapter of life during which your weight will take care of itself as long as you do a few things to maintain your metabolism. This chapter will show you how to do that.

WHAT DOES "UNPROCESSED" MEAN?

No doubt you have been advised to eat whole foods or unprocessed foods—they keep your metabolism humming along nicely. But what exactly does that mean? Apart from the wild berry plucked and eaten mid-stride on a hike, all food must be processed in some way. Is a peeled orange a whole food?

Researchers have proposed different definitions for this term, and some take into account the interests of food manufacturers and have no bearing on your health. The food categorization system that is most respected and that considers what matters most to our health comes from the work of Dr. Carlos Monteiro.

Dr. Monteiro has proposed three food groups: minimally processed, processed, and ultra-processed. In developing his groups, the diets of several different populations were evaluated in terms of what percentage of the diet comes from which group. When considered under real-world conditions, his model holds up and the conclusion is clear: the more unprocessed food, by Dr. Monteiro's definition, that a person eats, the less prone he or she will be to obesity and chronic disease.[1]

UNPROCESSED FOODS

Dr. Monteiro originally called these "minimally processed" foods. These foods have had the least possible modification to their original state in order to make them edible. The processing methods involved include cleaning, sprouting, chilling, fermenting, squeezing, fat reduction, wrapping, freezing, vacuum-packing, drying, and pasteurizing. These foods generally have a short shelf life, and they usually require further preparation before eating.

Unprocessed foods include:

- Fresh and frozen fruit
- Fresh and frozen vegetables
- Intact whole grains and nonflour grain fractions, such as steel-cut oats, bulgur wheat, and corn grits
- Whole and pureed beans and legumes, such as lentils beans, black beans, and pinto beans
- Raw shelled nuts and seeds
- Unflavored whole, low-fat, and nonfat milk, yogurt, and cottage cheese
- Eggs and egg whites
- Fresh and frozen poultry
- Fresh and frozen meat
- Fresh and frozen seafood and shellfish
- Naturally fermented foods mixed only with salt, herbs, and spices; examples include miso, kimchi, tempeh, sauerkraut, and chutney

- Culinary herbs and spices in their natural state, freeze-dried, or ground; examples include ginger, turmeric, garlic, cumin, black pepper, and salt without chemical additives

Unprocessed foods have no drawbacks—the more you build your diet on them, the better. Yes, it is possible to consume too much of them, but not probable. These foods are all pretty filling. When is the last time you snuck into the kitchen at night to finish off the leftover kale? They just are not the foods that lend themselves to overeating or mindless grazing. Their fuel content is low enough that the time it takes to eat them is usually slow enough so that you can feel full when you have had enough. Nuts may be the one exception—if they are used as a snack food, it is possible to overdo it.

PROCESSED FOODS

These include foods extracted from unprocessed foods. They are extracted to concentrate certain parts of the food or to extend the shelf life. These foods are processed by milling, refining, hydrogenation, or hydrolysis. Enzymes or additives may be used. Most of them are not eaten alone but, rather, are used as ingredients, often along with unprocessed foods. Although these are single-ingredient foods, they have a greater fuel density than the foods from which they are derived.

When used mindfully, processed foods can be part of a healthy diet. However, for many people, they can be culprits causing weight gain and chronic disease. They are less filling than unprocessed foods are. By this definition, processed foods probably will not make you crave them if you are not already hungry. Once you are eating them, however, it is easy to eat them well past the point of being comfortable. Their fuel density is high enough so that it is possible to eat too much of them before you know you're full. Unlike the next category, the highly processed foods, processed foods are less apt to trigger cravings when you are not even hungry, but they are easy to overconsume during meal time.

A simple rule is to allow yourself an extra serving of unprocessed foods, especially vegetables, but avoid extra servings of processed foods, such as:

- Butter
- Cheese
- Cream
- Corn syrup
- Dried fruits
- Gluten-containing flour and all flour products
- Gluten-free flour and all gluten-free flour products
- Lactose
- Lard
- Margarine
- Milk protein extracts
- Noodles and pasta
- Sugar
- Sweeteners, including honey, molasses, maple syrup
- Unsweetened breakfast cereals
- Vegetable oils

HIGHLY PROCESSED FOODS

These are usually a mixture of unprocessed and processed foods. They also have a long shelf life. They may be processed by baking, frying, or deep-frying. Many also have nonfood chemical additives, flavor enhancers, and preservatives—ick!

Highly processed foods have a strong tendency to trigger the brain's reward centers and alter the taste buds, making consumers come to prefer them. You've heard their tagline, "Bet you can't eat just one!" They are also the least apt to fill you up, especially those in liquid form. After eating them, many of us are still just as hungry and end up eating more than we need.

Those who are in excellent health are not harmed by having some of these foods on occasion. However, those who suffer from adiposity are best off just avoiding them as much as possible. Many find that when they completely avoid these foods, their appetite becomes much more manageable. Examples include:

- Bacon
- Biscuits
- Breads
- Cakes

- Candy
- Canned soups
- Cereal bars
- Cheesecake
- Chicken nuggets
- Cookies
- Deli meats
- Donuts
- Fast food
- Fish sticks
- French fries
- Fried chicken
- Frozen pizzas
- Hot dogs
- Ice cream
- Pastries
- Potato chips
- Sauces
- Sausage
- Smoked and cured meats
- Soda
- Sweetened beverages
- Tortilla chips

During the Reset phase, you focused your diet on unprocessed foods and avoided highly processed foods. Many people with strong food cravings and food addiction find it is easier to eliminate the highly processed foods completely than it is to reduce them. Of course, this advice is still sound after the Reset phase, but most find that when their livers are healthier, they are less apt to be thrown into a cycle of cravings by small deviations.

EAT LOTS OF FOOD CATEGORIES

Like most narratives, it seems that fad diets need to have a villain. These fad diets contradict each other about what is the true villain food, but they are in complete agreement that all our maladies are the result of one particular heinous food villain. Scary!

So, people usually eschew the villain after being educated about its maliciousness. Then, they are rewarded with all things good—weight loss, vibrant health, and the confidence of knowing they have found the truth. This process takes a few days to start and usually lasts anywhere from a few weeks to a year or so at the most. But then the benefits seem to dwindle, so people double down. Whatever that villain is, they must not be avoiding it enough. They suspect some hidden sources, or perhaps it is more powerful than they imagined and even the little bits thought to be harmless are enough to take away that promised salvation. After that, a new cycle begins, although it will likely last less than half as long as the first. It becomes obvious that the concept is no longer working, and they surrender, abandoning the diet. They have given in to the food villain and pay dearly for it.

At that point, people resume eating more or less what they did before they had begun the diet. They edit their memory to believe the diet was sound but that they had failed.

Nearly all the reasoning behind "villain" diets is based on thought experiments, test-tube studies, or animal tests—all with questionable relevance to humans. The other approach is to hold up the examples of people who have had valid, but uncommon, reactions to certain foods. Just because someone can have a bad reaction to a particular food does not mean it is bad for everyone. I'm terribly allergic to horse dander, yet that does not mean that equestrian pursuits are bad ideas for everyone.

Mind you, some people are harmed by certain foods. Others have dramatic anaphylactic allergies, like to peanuts, or longstanding reactions to gluten in the case of celiac or to lactose in the case of lactose intolerance, and still others have intolerances and sensitivities that may come and go. If you suspect a personal reaction to certain foods, work with your healthcare provider to pinpoint which foods are the culprits and whether you can reverse the reactions. Most sensitivities and intolerances are reversible.

As omnivores, we can subsist on a bewildering variety of foods. And the broader the range of our diet is, the more we thrive. When we cut out whole categories of food from our diets, we start to lose the ability to tolerate those particular foods. The more categories we remove, the less diverse our flora becomes. The ensuing cycles involve real but new food intolerances, risks for micronutrient deficiencies, and lost opportunities from the benefit of phytonutrients.

If you have fallen into the "food villain" trap, there is still hope. Start with tiny amounts and find a few foods in each category that you do well with. Each time you shop, find a food you've not had for a while and slowly keep expanding your menu.

EAT FOR SATIETY

The more your diet comprises unprocessed foods, the more you will fill up on the least amount of food. If you want to really be strategic about this, search out the data showing that, within the category of unprocessed foods, some are more filling than others. This was shown to be true in a study called the *Satiety Index of Common Foods* that was led by Dr. Susanne Holt. To date, this is the only published study that tested the concept and found out how satisfying various foods really are.

In the study, volunteers were fed 38 different foods. They were given each food in a controlled portion that equaled 240 calories, served beneath a light-blocking hood to reduce the possible effects of the food's visual appeal and eaten in roughly the same-sized bites and at the same temperature. After each food was consumed, the researchers asked the volunteers to rate their hunger levels. Two hours later, they were allowed to eat any food they wanted, in any quantity they chose, from a buffet. They could go back for as much as they wanted. The scientists worked behind the scenes to measure exactly how much food each participant ate. They also tracked their hunger levels afterward (every 15 minutes).

Here is how they scored it. If a 240-calorie snack made the participants feel full and caused them to eat less at the buffet, then that snack was considered satisfying. If another 240-calorie snack left them hungry and they ate more food afterward, it was considered less satisfying. White bread was given an arbitrary score of 100 and other foods were ranked accordingly, based on how filling it was compared to it.

Some general concepts emerged. Fiber, protein, water, and starch were the most filling, whereas sugar and fat were the least filling. Croissants were the single least filling food in the study, followed closely by cake, with scores of 47 and 65, respectively. Boiled potatoes were the most filling food per calorie by far, with a score of 323. (It is no coincidence they are the highest food source of resistant starch.) The second most filling food was codfish at 225, followed by oatmeal at 209.

Potatoes make a great case study for the power of food processing. In the Holt study mentioned on page 217, boiled potatoes were the most filling food. Other studies have looked at
the maximum calorie density per weight of foods, while others
have explored how much a particular food in one's diet predicts
weight gain.

As luck would have it, those studies independently have all
settled on the same food as the worst: potato chips. So, are
potatoes good or bad? It is all about the processing. When cut
and boiled, potatoes are one of the best foods you will find.
When they are spray-dried, chemically treated, mill-rolled, and
deep-fried, they are the worst.

Here are the less-processed foods from the study in the
order of most filling to least filling:

- Boiled potatoes—323
- Codfish—225
- Oatmeal—209
- Oranges—202
- Apples—197
- Brown pasta—188
- Beef—176
- Baked beans—168
- Grapes—162
- Whole-grain bread—157
- Popcorn—154
- Bran cereal—151
- Eggs—150
- Cheese—147
- Lentils—133
- Brown rice—132
- Bananas—118
- Muesli—100
- Yogurt (flavored)—88
- Peanuts—84

If you struggle with hunger, focus on unprocessed foods
and make boiled potatoes and oatmeal your daily staples.[2]

EAT YOUR VEGGIES

There never was a debate: veggies offer lots of helpful nutrients that most
of us do not get enough of. Veggies help us in three main ways. One way

is that they directly supply essential vitamins and minerals needed for all the body's metabolic reactions. Many of these, like folate, vitamin K, magnesium, potassium, beta-carotene, and vitamin C, are rarely found in low-vegetable diets.

The second way they help is that they have phytonutrients that feed the bowel flora. Scientists understand that the flora is healthiest when diets contain lots of different vegetables and fruits. These phytonutrients work collectively in ways that we are just barely starting to appreciate. Some of the active phytonutrients found in veggies include catechins, lycopene, luteolin, sulforaphane, ellagic acid, flavonoids, phytoestrogens, glucosinolates, and polyphenols.

The simplest way to cover all the bases is to have at least one vegetable from each of the following groups every day:

- Leafy greens—spinach, chard, kale, romaine, collards
- Cruciferous—broccoli, Brussels sprouts, bok choy, cabbage, arugula
- Allium—onions, garlic, leeks, scallions, shallots
- Apiaceae—carrots, celery, parsnips, parsley, cilantro
- Edible fungi—button mushrooms, shiitake, enoki, portobello, oyster mushrooms

To get enough veggies, make your lunch and dinner about half vegetables by food volume.

EAT FOR FIBER DIVERSITY

Your bowel flora help everything to work better. And the flora need variety to stay healthy just as much as you do. They feed on fibers and they come in many types. In fact, do not think of fiber as a single thing; fiber comprises a broad range of things. Following are some the most important categories of fiber, what they help with, and which foods they are in.

When you see all these diverse types of fiber and their benefits, you understand why the best diets embrace the widest range of foods. Low carb and paleo diets can supply only 10 of the 17 types of essential fiber.

Ketogenic diets supply 4 of the 17 at most. In short, diets that exclude entire food categories inevitably lead to a less diverse and resilient bowel flora. The diet that will give you the best metabolism will include intact whole grains, legumes, nuts, fungi, vegetables, seeds, tubers, and fruits.

Fiber type	Food categories	Specific foods	Benefits
Cellulose	Fruits, vegetables, legumes, grains, nuts, seeds	Apples, bananas, raspberries, carrots, beets, broccoli, collard greens, spinach, artichokes Black beans, navy beans, pinto beans, garbanzo beans Almonds, pumpkin seeds, flaxseeds, walnuts	Increases the length of the colon, associated with protection against DSS. Dietary fibers have been observed to decrease colitis severity in acute and chronic rodent models.
Hemicelluloses (hexose, pentose)	Whole grains	Steel-cut oats, oat bran, rice bran, wheat bran	Increase bowel regularity and hydration, reduce cholesterol absorption.
Lignin	Root vegetables, berry seeds	Flaxseeds, sesame seeds	May improve gut integrity, may reduce the risk of cancer, antioxidant properties.
Pectin	Apples, citrus fruits, legumes, nuts	Citrus peels, navel oranges, Braeburn apples, Gala apples, dried apricots	Apple pectin has cholesterol-lowering properties in rats and decreases total cholesterol levels in humans. Contradictory studies on pectin report no effect on cholesterol levels.
Hydrocolloids (gums)	Natural thickening agents	Xanthan gum, guar gum, gum Arabic, acacia gum, carboxymethyl cellulose, Agar-agar, glucomannan—konjac root	Cholesterol-lowering properties, reduced adiposity and hepatic steatosis, relief of abdominal pain in patients with irritable bowel syndrome.

Fiber type	Food categories	Specific foods	Benefits
Oat beta glucan	Oats, barley, rye	Gluten-free rolled oats, steel-cut oats, whole oats, oat bran, pearled barley, whole-grain rye	LDL reduction up to 16.5%, lower postprandial blood glucose, improved wound healing.
Mushroom beta glucan	Dietary and medicinal mushrooms	Common white mushrooms, Reishi, shiitake, chaga, maitake, cremini, sclerotia	Anticarcinogenic, antiviral, immunomodulatory, lower IL-4 and IL-5 cytokines, increased IL-12, decreases in post-surgical infections.
Inulin	Certain root vegetables	Dandelion root, chicory root, Jerusalem artichokes	Reduced tumor incidence initiated by carcinogenic compounds such as azoxymethane (AOM) and dimethylhydrazine. Lowers plasma triacylglycerol.
Fructo-oligosaccharides (FOS, fructans)	Certain vegetables and fruits	Onion, chicory, garlic, asparagus, banana, artichokes, and other vegetables	May prevent colorectal cancer. Associated with reduced mucosal inflammation and lesion scores in a rat model of colitis, reduction in body weight in human subjects, promotes satiety, increases IL-10 production in intestinal dendritic cells in Crohn's disease patients.
Galacto-oligosaccharides (GOS, galactans)	Legumes	Lentils, garbanzo beans, green peas, lima beans, kidney beans	Improve blood sugar, lower cholesterol, improve liver function. May play a role in prevention or progression of colorectal cancer. Increased calcium absorption, may improve IBS symptoms.

Fiber type	Food categories	Specific foods	Benefits
Raffinose Oligosaccharides (ROS, raffinose)	Legumes	Black-eyed peas, lima beans, kidney beans	Lower risk of gram-negative bacterial infections and yeast overgrowth.
Stachyose, verbascose	Cruciferous vegetables	Cabbage, Brussels sprouts, broccoli, asparagus	Alleviation of constipation, improved hormone conversion.
Resistant starch—RS1	Seeds or legumes and unprocessed whole grains, coarsely milled grains, seeds or legumes	Cracked wheat, red beans, raw steel-cut oats, pinto beans, white beans	Decreases risk of colorectal cancer by increasing SCFA, decrease in fecal pH and transit time, increased insulin sensitivity.
Resistant starch—RS2	High amylopectin pea starch, high amylose corn starch, raw potato, unripe banana	RS2 Pea starch in original Reset Shake (see page 119), green banana flour, unmodified potato starch	Reduces hunger, improves weight loss, lowers glucose levels, increases metabolism of fat, increases GLP1.
Resistant starch—RS3	Cooled potato, rice, pasta	Boiled and refrigerated potatoes, chilled sushi rice	Improve basal metabolic rate, improve bowel flora.
Mannitol	Variety of plants and fungi	Watermelon, mushrooms, cauliflower, celery, sweet potatoes	Increased calcium and magnesium absorption and retention.
Sorbitol	Variety of plants	Apples, pears, peaches, prunes	Prevents diet-induced obesity, improves calcium absorption.

DON'T OVERFILL YOUR FUEL TANK

You know the whole debate about what we should eat to stay lean: fats, ketones, or carbs? Your liver cannot tell the difference. Too much fuel clogs it and hurts it, no matter where it comes from.

The best diet is not defined by what you avoid. It is defined by how well you provide your body *with* unprocessed foods without overloading your fuel storage. So how do you meet your fuel needs?

EAT OPTIMAL PROTEIN

Calories come from fuel and protein. As explained earlier, you will stay most lean when you get an optimal intake of about a gram of protein for every pound of body weight. For most people, this means that protein takes up about one-fourth to one-third of their calories. The rest must come from primarily a combination of fat and carbs.

This amount of protein is higher than the amount needed to ward off protein-deficiency diseases. To get it, it does take at least three daily servings of foods that contain over 20 grams of protein per serving. The advantages of optimal-protein diets include more effective detoxification, easier fat loss, less appetite, higher metabolic rate, and better muscle growth.

Quality protein can be found in selected vegetable sources, dairy foods, eggs, seafood, poultry, and meat. A variety of sources is best, but those who have chosen to avoid categories of protein foods can still meet their needs. For example, to meet your optimal protein needs, have a protein shake for breakfast and a serving of a protein-dense food for lunch and dinner.

Breakfast is a unique meal. Shakes are the best option because they supply a full 23 to 35 grams of protein and are quick to make. Many "protein-rich" breakfast foods don't actually contain that much protein. Two eggs are only 12 grams. Sausage or bacon will rarely give over 8 grams per serving. Cereal and milk usually have just 9 grams of protein.

Along with containing quality protein, shakes make it easy to get resistant starch and other quality fibers. So, you continue with shakes for breakfast and build your lunch and dinner around three elements: protein, fuel, and veggies.

EAT HEALTHY FATS

Like all other parts of the diet, fats are neither poisons to avoid nor magic elixirs to consume at any quantity. Fats contain essential fatty acids that we cannot produce in our bodies. Of these, omega-6 is easy to find, and nearly every source of fat contains it. Any diet that includes as little as a single handful of nuts and seeds per day as its source of fat will likely supply adequate omega-6 fats.

Omega-3 fats are found in fewer foods, so becoming deficient in them is more likely. There are three subtypes of omega-3s and each seems to be important: ALA, EPA, and DHA. Plant sources of omega-3 like flax, hemp, chia, and canola are rich in ALA. Most vegans and vegetarians who eat these foods can easily get enough ALA, and can usually convert it into EPA. If their diets are low in omega-6 foods, they may also be able to convert the ALA into DHA. However, vegans and vegetarians whose diets have higher fats become deficient in DHA because omega-6 can overwork the enzyme that turns ALA into DHA. Vegans can do fine on DHA if they lower their omega-6 intake or add an algae-derived DHA supplement. Those who eat fish or seafood several times per week get plenty of EPA and DHA, but they should still consume plant-derived sources of ALA.

Once the need for essential fats has been met, fats can easily become a source of unnecessary extra fuel. This is especially true for processed versions of fat like vegetable oils, butter, margarine, bacon, ice cream, and lard. Unfortunately, many experts have confused helpful fats with essential fats. There are many fats your body uses for essential reactions like the repair of brain cells or the production of hormones. In fact, some of these roles are so helpful that evolution has given our bodies the ability to make fats like saturated fat and cholesterol whenever we need them—that is why they are not classified as essential fats.

Since we make these fats naturally, it's not necessary to get them from outside sources. And because foods that contain them, like butter, lard, or red meat, are so dense in fuel, they become empty fuel sources.

If your goal is to stay lean, ward off chronic disease, and keep your brain healthy, your approach to fats is simple. Each day, include minimally processed fats from a variety of sources; have between one and three servings of unprocessed fats such as:

- Almonds
- Avocados
- Chia seeds
- Salmon
- Flaxseed
- Walnuts
- Sunflower seeds

At least twice weekly, include seafood or high sources of plant omega-3 like flaxseeds. Do not use nuts or seeds as snacks. Similarly, avoid processed fats like oil, butter, and margarine as much as possible. The single oil with the largest body of positive evidence is extra-virgin olive oil. Use it as your main oil, but use it sparingly and keep the temperatures low when cooking with it.

The heat-stable oil with the largest amount of health-promoting evidence based on over 270 human studies is canola oil.[3] Many health experts have warned about its dangers, however. The concerns about erucic acid are not relevant, since modern canola oil contains no more of it than other cruciferous vegetables do.[4] The concerns about GMO and solvent extraction are valid, as they are for oils. So, select organic, expeller-pressed non-GMO forms of canola oil and, like any other oil, use it sparingly. Use a home sprayer or brush it on lightly when greasing a pan for sautéing.

EAT GOOD CARBS

How public experts feel about carbs at any given point is predictably the opposite of how they feel about fats. These two nutrients are rightfully linked because both are main fuel sources. If a diet encourages you to restrict one, by default it allows you to consume the other more freely. Both are important parts of the diet, yet both can be overdone.

Unlike fats, carbs do not contain any nutrients that our bodies cannot synthesize. There are no "essential" carbs. However, this does not mean you need to avoid carbs completely or that they are innately unhealthy. Food components can be important and helpful without falling under the category of "essential."

Most of the public is now aware that healthy bowel flora are necessary for good body size, strong immune system, and quick brain function. Carbs are to your bowel flora what water is to a garden. Fats, ketones, and alcohol have no positive effects on the bowel flora—only carbs do.

As we've discussed, resistant starch is, to date, the best-documented food ingredient for improving the types of flora that lower cancer risk, improve fat burning, and stabilize blood sugar. The foods highest in resistant starch include boiled potatoes, legumes, and plantains. So, each day include two to three servings of unprocessed carbs, such as:

- Boiled potatoes
- Sweet potatoes
- Yams
- Steel-cut oats
- Buckwheat porridge
- Bulgur wheat

- Brown rice
- Pinto beans
- Black beans
- Lentils
- Kabocha squash
- Parsnips

Try to have at least one of them be from a high-RS food like legumes or potatoes, or include an RS supplement.

SHOULD YOU FAVOR FATS OR CARBS?

I would like to discourage you from identifying your diet as either low-fat or low-carb. Studies have shown that either approach can cause fat loss, but only if there is a reduction in total fuel intake. Either approach works for a while because, when you cut down on either fats or carbs, you also reduce fuel intake.[5] The drawbacks to going low on either are that you can (1) get low in essential nutrients and (2) get bored owing to having fewer food options.

So, have one serving of fuel total for each meal. That would be one serving of carbs, or one serving of fats, or, as an occasional option, one serving of wine. For example, you could have a salmon salad for lunch with salmon as the protein, romaine lettuce as the veggie, and extra-virgin olive oil as the fuel. On another day, you could make a sandwich of sprouted-grain bread as the fuel, homemade shredded chicken as the protein, and butter lettuce, sliced tomatoes, sliced red onion, and broccoli sprouts for the veggies.

A dinner could have a "pasta" entree with zucchini noodles, a sauce of simmered tomatoes for the veggie, and lightly sautéed tempeh with extra-virgin olive oil for the protein and fuel. On a special occasion, you might choose wine for your fuel with dinner and serve it with sautéed scallops for protein and steamed spinach for the veggie.

I suggest limiting your alcohol to wine and beer, and consuming no more than a few servings per week total. In the past, many thought that one or two servings of alcohol per day could result in health benefits, but now we know that this was based on misleading information. People who do not drink may appear less healthy than light drinkers only if you ignore the fact that many who avoid alcohol do so for medical reasons that directly affect their health. For example, some people who do not drink have a history of alcoholism, liver disease, or are on medications that are not safe to mix with alcohol. However, when you compare the health of those who do not drink by choice against that of light and moderate drinkers, those who do not drink by choice have the lowest rates of mortality.[6]

DON'T SNACK ON FUEL

Most people will do well to avoid snacking as a habit. It is a recent habit, and people in the parts of the world that have adopted it are the ones with the obesity crisis.

There was a time when many thought that frequent meals helped fat loss. We now know that idea does not stand up to scrutiny. By keeping your liver healthy and eating solid meals, you will likely find that you do not need to eat as often.

If you do feel hungry between meals, take a look at your unlimited food options. Just like during the Reset phase, these are great options for anytime you like. The other option is to save some of your meal until later. Say, if mid-afternoon is when you start to feel hungry, just set aside some of your lunch and leave it until then.

This strategy works even better when you use some unlimited foods to stretch your lunch out further. For example, suppose your lunch was salmon for protein, brown rice for fuel, and 1 cup of broccoli for veggie. You could package up one-third each of the salmon and rice, add an extra cup of broccoli, and set it aside to eat as a mid-afternoon snack.

EXERCISE

We learned that in the case of the adiposity, the liver has lost its ability to store any extra fuel. When your liver is unclogged, it is able to recruit your muscles as an extra place to store any spare fuel. There is a special glucose receptor in your muscles called glut-4 that is largely responsible for the muscles' ability to take up and store fuel.

Imagine muscle and body fat as people in line at a cafeteria. When glut-4 is active, muscle cuts to the front of the line and gets all the food. Thus, the key to healthy glut-4 receptors is exercise. The more your exercise varies in type, duration, and intensity, the more fuel-hungry your muscles get.

EXERCISE FOR MAINTENANCE

Since during the Reset phase, you limit exercise to walks and micro workouts, what now works best for the Maintenance phase?

Toward the goal of keeping your metabolism healthy, plan on doing some version of exercise every day. Many experts encourage exercising a few days per week—mostly because they are afraid that if they encourage more, no one will exercise at all. I have found that planning for three to five days per week often ends up translating into three to five days per month. Just think of exercise as a daily habit, and plan your days accordingly. Once you get into a routine and have that habit in place, it is much easier to stick with. If for some reason you miss a day, dust yourself off and get back on track—no worries. Pick it up again as a daily habit and think about a way to work around whatever threw you off the next time that comes up.

Some days this routine can be pretty easy. If you are rundown or crunched for time, just do a casual walk or a restorative yoga session. Give yourself a minimum target of 30 minutes of movement of some sort.

When you are healthy and your metabolism is working well, do not be surprised if exercise becomes a healthy addiction. The dangers of over-training or chronic cardio are real, but the people at true risk are the weekend warriors—those who are sedentary all week and then do high-intensity, prolonged activities for many hours during the weekend. It is normal to have more time for fun on the weekend, but just keep active during the week so your body can accommodate it.

The main benefits of exercise include a better mood, a healthier metabolism, lower risk of chronic disease, better sleep, and better brain function. These benefits start to show up with as little as 20 minutes exercise per day. And they get really exciting at 40 minutes per day, and then they keep getting better up to about 90 minutes per day. When does regular exercise get harmful? In a group of 600,000 adults, 200 minutes per day did not seem to show any signs of causing harm.[7]

Once you get some momentum, include a mixture of strength training, flexibility training, agility and balance activities, low-intensity cardio, and high-intensity cardio.

Remember, most of us spend several hours per evening in nonessential media time, whether it is TV, social media, games, or just web browsing. If you cut this time in half, you can do some physical activity before dinner and still get to bed early enough so that you can wake up in time to exercise.

What does the ultimate exercise schedule look like? Assuming your goal is general health and performance, as opposed to a specific type of athletic competition, it could look like the following table.

DAY	ACTIVITIES		
	Morning	**Evening**	**Before bed**
Monday	Walk 10k steps	10-minute intervals	5 minutes of stretching
Tuesday	30-minute run	15-minute calisthenics	5 minutes of stretching
Wednesday	30 minutes weights in gym	Recreational tennis	5 minutes of stretching
Thursday	Spin class	Bike ride around neighborhood	5 minutes of stretching
Friday	Yoga class	Walk 10k steps	5 minutes of stretching
Saturday	2-hour hike	Projects around the home	5 minutes of stretching
Sunday	Long session in the gym	Projects in the yard	5 minutes of stretching

DON'T SIT STILL

You may have heard taglines like "sitting is the new smoking." It seems that prolonged immobility may negate the benefits of exercise. If your work is sedentary, find some method that allows you to move for 5 to 10 minutes of every hour.

One of the simplest ways is through optimal hydration. When you continue your habit of drinking 8 glasses of water, you will have an automatic movement reminder built into your bladder. You can also use any of the numerous fitness trackers. I've used Apple watches and Garmin watches. Both nagged me to move if I sat still more than 50 minutes at a time. You can also use a simple hourly chime on a watch or clock or an egg-timer. Each hour, walk at least 100 steps and if you can, do a few shoulder circles and neck rotations.

Nothing in this chapter was too hard, too weird, or too extreme, was it? Once you complete your Reset, these basic habits will help you stay thin and energized without needing to diet.

chapter ten

FAQ

It is hard to give the same advice to different people. Your health is a function of the unique intersection of your lineage, societal forces, upbringing, genetics, hormonal patterns, beliefs, peers, and random luck. The steps that helped someone else regain his health might require some modification or clarification for your situation.

Thankfully, we are alike in far more ways than we are different, and the differences that do exist fall into predictable patterns. After guiding tens of thousands of people through this Reset process, my team and I have built this program in a way that answers most questions before they get asked. Nonetheless, there are some important questions that come up often enough that they are worth addressing directly.

If your question is not among these here, or it is not answered in enough detail, please do not despair. Visit the Metabolism Reset support group at metabolismresetdietbook.com/support. You can search through hundreds of questions and ask your own questions directly. Between our community, my team, and myself, you are sure to get a good answer in short order.

SPECIAL CIRCUMSTANCES

MENOPAUSE

Will the Reset program work if I am in or near menopause?

Yes. Not only can it work, it may be the best option. Many women have experienced sudden onset mid-body weight gain around menopause that seems not to respond to any level of effort.

In menopause, the metabolism changes because the liver also goes through corresponding changes.[1] In fact, some have called this process "hepatopause."

Medicine defines menopause as having no periods for a year. The average woman has her last period at age 50 years and 3 months. However, there's large variation in this age indicator, which can be normal. *Perimenopause* is defined as menstrual irregularities or symptoms like hot flashes that start in the years leading up to menopause. Most women have some signs of perimenopause by the time they are in their mid-40s.

During perimenopause, estrogen levels may jump up and down. If a woman is prone to gain weight, these changes can cause weight gain to be concentrated in parts of the body where adipose tissues have the most estrogen receptors—the hips, thighs, and breasts. When a woman loses weight, these areas may be the last to show it. In both perimenopause and menopause, women often have a decline in androgenic hormones like testosterone and DHEA. This hormone drop makes them more prone to losing muscle tissue, especially while dieting.[2]

In later stages of menopause, estrogen levels get lower, making collagen repair less effective. The loss of collagen can cause cellulite and loose skin. It can make women also less able to form subcutaneous fat. That might sound like a good thing, but it is not. When subcutaneous fat cells cannot grow, they are more apt to send spare fuel to get stored in more dangerous places, like around the organs.

The good news is that not only can the Reset program still work but, because of how it works, it may be the best option for women near menopausal age. By providing abundant amounts of fiber and RS, the program will help the liver and the bowel flora buffer the normal hormonal changes. By keeping the muscles stimulated through optimal protein and micro workouts, it can prevent the muscle loss that leads to weight regain. Finally, by providing phytonutrients and improving the liver's phase 2 efficiency, many women notice that hot flashes and night sweats are greatly reduced during the program.

VEGAN

Can I do the Reset if I am vegetarian or vegan?

Yes, you can. Vegans and vegetarians do not have to worry about getting a protein deficiency (see more on pages 14 and 32). Do consider that when your fuel intake is low, as it is during the Reset, your body can easily break down lots of muscle tissue, setting you up to gain more weight than you lost. To prevent that, the Reset program provides a gram of protein for each pound of body weight. This is easy to do on a vegetarian diet, but takes a bit more planning when you factor in the fact that you are limiting carbs and fats. Many foods have protein and can prevent a protein deficiency, but they are not dense in protein and cannot help you get to an optimal level of a low-fuel diet. For people of all diets, we have far fewer food options for dense protein than we do for fats, carbs, or veggies.

Beans are wonderful sources of protein, but if you rely on them as your main protein source during the Reset, you will get too much fuel from carbs. Likewise, nuts, seeds, and cheese also have protein, but if you eat enough of them to meet your protein needs, you will go way over your target for dietary fat.

If you are vegan, your best protein-dense foods include vegetable protein powder, tempeh, tofu, edamame, and seitan. If you are vegetarian, you can also include eggs, egg whites, cottage cheese, Icelandic yogurt, and Greek yogurt; choose nonfat and unsweetened for both types of yogurt.

If you avoid animal foods for health reasons, consider that most pioneers of the modern vegetarian movements, including John Robins[3] and Joel Fuhrman,[4] have now acknowledged that consciously sourced seafood can provide more benefits than detriments. Other vegan leaders like John Mackay[5] have acknowledged that you get the same health benefits if you include up to 10 percent of calories from consciously selected animal foods.

There are also many who are vegans who have consciously chosen to eat mollusks.[6] Oysters, clams, and mussels lack the requisite neurologic apparatus required to experience suffering. They also can have a net positive impact on the environment when grown correctly. Furthermore, as rich sources of EPA, DHA, vitamin B_{12}, iron, and zinc, they have a perfect complement of nutrients that may be lacking in a plant-based diet.

NIGHT SHIFT

Can I do the Reset if I work the night shift?

Yes, and here are some strategies to use. Sleep is one of the most important parts of metabolic flexibility. It seems that your daily circadian rhythm is woven into your body's ability to burn stored fat for fuel. You can get healthier if you work the night shift, but it does take a bit more planning.

On the days you work, the goal is to simulate a normal day's schedule as much as possible. For example, say you work from 10 p.m. to 6 a.m.; here is how you would schedule your day to maintain your circadian rhythm: When you finish work at 6 a.m., you want to treat your next few hours as your evening. Have your solid meal at this time. You need to allow for several hours to wind down from your workday so that you can get some sleep. During the last hour before bedtime, darken your home as much as possible. It is worth investing in tools like blackout shades and a comfortable sleep mask. It also helps to have a lamp with a red bulb or amber-colored glasses to mimic the light patterns of dusk. Also, try to avoid all display screens during this last hour.

Choose a place to sleep where you will not be disturbed, and aim for a full eight hours of sleep. In our example, you could sleep from 10 a.m. to 6 p.m. When you wake up, expose yourself to bright lights. If it is still daylight outdoors, spend at least 30 minutes outside during your first waking hour and have your breakfast shake at this same time. If it is no longer daylight when you wake up, consider investing in SAD lights.

Time your lunch shake to be equidistant between your breakfast and dinner. For example, if you have your first meal when you wake up at 7 p.m. and your last meal at 7 a.m. before bedtime, have your lunch shake near 2 a.m. while you are at work. You are still welcome to have unlimited foods as needed for snacks at other times if hunger becomes too intense.

If you work three nights per week or fewer, keep a normal schedule on your days off. If you work four or more nights, keep to the modified night schedule above even on your days off.

TRAVELING

Can I do the Reset when I'm traveling during part of it?

Yes, in fact, many people have told me they were surprised to find that traveling is one of the easiest times to do a Reset. Much of the stress from traveling comes from trying to find good food. Once you get the hang of the pre-made meal-replacement options in Chapters 4 and 5, you may find yourself using them just to make travel more convenient.

All you do is pack each dry serving of shake into a small storage bag and pack them all into your shaker bottle—do not add liquid. You can carry this combo in checked or carry-on luggage. When you go through carry-on, security may stop and visually inspect it. My wife and I often leave our bags open with the shake set-up visible to save them time.

Your one main meal is not too hard to do in restaurants. Start with a large mixed salad or steamed veggies. Be sure to have them hold the oil, croutons, cheese, and dressing. Then add a lean protein such as fish, poultry, lean meat, or tempeh. And have some good carbs. When eating out, baked potatoes, bean dishes, or brown rice are often easiest to find.

Your micro workouts are perfect for doing on the road, since you do not need any equipment for them anyway. It seems odd to say, but the one pitfall can be walking too much. If you end up covering over 20,000 steps in a day, you may wish to add one extra serving of your shake. Just know that if this becomes a daily strategy, your Reset will be less effective.

MAJOR HOLIDAYS

What if my Reset coincides with one of the big holidays?

Avoid overlap between the first few days and major holidays, if possible. If you are doing a Reset over a holiday season and you will be attending a holiday party, your best option is to focus on lean protein and extra veggies at the holiday meal. Good carbs are the hardest part of a Reset meal to find when eating at parties. Remember that just because it is the holiday season, that does not mean you need to change your daily habits. As long as you can negotiate the holiday events, you can keep your days the same as you would otherwise.

AIP

Can I do the Reset if I'm on an Autoimmune Paleo diet?

No problem! You can still do the Metabolism Reset just fine. You have a shorter list of resistant starch (RS) foods to choose from, and you will be avoiding nightshades, but neither of these adaptations are difficult.

Bear in mind that there is no one universal Autoimmune Paleo (AIP) food list, but the suggestions that follow do adhere to most. Another general consideration is that none of the proponents of AIP recommend it as a long-term diet. All nutrition experts agree that healthy diets do not eliminate large numbers of food categories forever. Also consider that many people have had relapses, as autoimmune diseases coincide with other dietary changes, including raw foods, vegan diets, Mediterranean diets, less strict paleo diets, and fat-free diets. Given that contradicting diets can lead to the same results prompts me to think that either the outcomes correlated with the diets, but were not caused by the diets; or they were caused by things the diets included, rather than things the diets excluded.

What do all of these diets include? High amounts of vegetables. Perhaps it is more about what you add in than what you leave out.

The main food categories excluded on AIP are grains, legumes, nuts, seeds, fungi, nightshade vegetables, and most vegetable oils. Here are some AIP-approved sources of critical nutrients for the Metabolism Reset.

Food category	AIP-approved options
RS	Green banana flour, plantains
Legumes	Snap peas, green beans and haricots verts (thin French green beans), green peas
Oils	Extra-virgin olive oil, avocado oil
Good Carbs	Sweet potatoes, turnips, parsnips, winter squash

Case Study: Sally

Sally learned about the Metabolism Reset diet online and thought it might help her digestive problems, with the added bonus of shedding a few extra pounds along the way. She had been on an Autoimmune Paleo protocol for the last several years. Although the diet was highly restrictive, it did seem to help lower thyroid antibodies at first. After she stayed on it, it seemed that her antibodies elevated again and she started gaining weight.

She also started having more issues with her digestion and had been diagnosed as having intestinal yeast overgrowth. Even though her diet was already limited, it seemed that the list of foods she could digest well was dwindling by the week.

Sally had seen several of my videos talking about resistant starch and wondered if part of her problem came from her very low intake of fiber and carbohydrate, so that she was starving her good bacteria. She started the program like a champ, exactly as directed. Knowing she was sensitive to many foods, she allowed herself one week on about half the recommended doses of resistant starch to let her body acclimate.

By the end of the four weeks, she barely even noticed the benefits to her waist because she was so excited about her stomach being flat—despite the fact that she was eating many foods she had not tolerated for months. A year after finishing her first Reset, her thyroid antibodies were at an all-time low and the range of foods in her diet was at an all-time high. Even though it seems that she could tolerate more foods, she still stuck to mostly unprocessed foods. She was feeling great, and was finally at the level of health she always felt was possible.

ABOUT THE DIET

CARBS

How can I lose weight while eating carbs? I thought carbs raised insulin and weight loss was impossible when insulin was high.

This idea is called the "carbohydrate hypothesis of obesity." The operating assumption behind it is that weight gain is solely the consequence of carbs raising insulin and insulin causing fat cells to grow. There is some truth in this concept, but not in its conclusions. In a bizarre counterexample, one of the best-studied diets for morbid obesity involved nothing but rice and fruit—all carbs. Because it is too restrictive, it is not a program I would advise, but it did work in its day. Duke University carefully documented roughly 18,000 cases of people cured of severe obesity, high blood pressure, diabetes, and even kidney failure.[7] If carbs and insulin were villains, this would not have worked.

Here are some details on why the carb hypothesis of obesity has been rejected: Carbs do raise insulin and insulin can promote the growth of fat cells. But there are a few problems with treating these statements as absolutes. Fat cells can grow from any excess of fuel, regardless of whether it is carbs, fats, or even ketones.[8] All fuel gets broken down into acetyl CoA (CoA). If the body needs the energy to burn, CoA gets burned. If the body's energy stores in the liver and muscles are low, CoA gets stored there. After the main stores are filled up, any extra gets stored as fat.

As for insulin, on a low-carb or ketogenic diet, you can gain weight just while having low insulin levels if your total fuel level is above your body's needs. Insulin does cause more carbs to enter your adipose cells, but it also causes more carbs to enter your liver and your muscle. When you need more fuel in these places and you just ate some carbs, that is appropriate. But what if you have too much fuel in your adipose cells or liver? Then your cells ignore insulin on purpose. This is called "insulin resistance" and it is a feature, not a glitch. Your body is keeping the fuel in circulation because it has nowhere to go. This effect also happens to fats as circulating triglycerides and even to ketones. When there is no room for fuel, your body resists it on purpose.

FAT ADAPTED

Don't I need to eat more fat to become a fat burner?

The thought is that if we eat lots of dietary fat, our bodies will enter into a chain reaction that will get out of control and burn up lots of adipose tissue. Many have thought that the simple act of eating more fat will make their bodies better at burning fat (adipose tissue). But the confusion is largely created by language. The phrase "burning fat" means two different things. Burning fat from the diet as fuel is called "beta-oxidation," whereas burning adipose tissue from the body's storage is a completely different process called "lipolysis."[9]

When your liver is blocked, both beta-oxidation and lipolysis are more difficult.[10] Remember, the core problem is that your liver cannot use fuel as quickly as it gets it, and it cannot burn stored triglycerides owing to a lack of glycogen. Any additional fuel you add in will just make the bottleneck that much worse. It does not matter if that fuel comes from carbs, dietary fats, or even from ketones—it is all fuel to your liver.[11]

Ironically, we cannot burn fat for fuel (beta-oxidation)

when our diet is too high in fat because beta-oxidation requires a compound called oxaloacetate (OAA), which is made only from carbs or protein. When someone eats more fat, yes, she does burn more fat—those fats that she ate. Studies have shown that when two groups of people eat the same number of calories and one group eats more fat, the high-fat group does burn more fat from their diets, while the lower fat group burns more fat from their bodies.[12]

KETOGENIC DIET

Don't I need to be on a ketogenic diet to lose weight?

First, let's distinguish metabolic ketosis from a ketogenic diet. Anytime your fuel intake gets low and you run out of glycogen, your liver can no longer burn body fat. It takes fat from the diet and turns it into ketones, which it cannot use, but other parts of the body can. This is metabolic ketosis and can occur on any low-fuel diet regardless of whether it is high or low in carbs, fats, or proteins. Metabolic ketosis produces mild amounts of ketones, and they can be useful since they might make someone feel less hungry and mentally foggy than he would otherwise.

In a ketogenic diet, carbs and proteins are limited and 80 percent or more of calories come from fat. Many advocate eating as much fat as needed to feel full, as long as carbs and protein are kept at a low enough level. In these cases, the body cannot burn fat for fuel, and so it is all converted into ketones. In advanced ketosis, there are also more ketones than the body can burn and ketone resistance sets in. This is the only circumstances in which ketones elevate to high levels in the urine or blood. They are there not because your body is burning ketones but, rather, because your body has too much fuel and it is rejecting ketones.

These circulating ketones are eventually converted into triglycerides and stored in the fat cells, just like excess carbs and fat can be. Studies have shown that ketogenic diets are even less effective at inducing fat loss than high-sugar diets, when they are matched for fuel.[13]

The Metabolism Reset diet does induce mild nutritional ketosis, which is part of why it gets easier after the first few days and also why a brief, more pronounced low fuel intake can be easier than prolonged but milder fuel deficit. The latter may not elicit the formation of appetite-suppressing ketones. However, it is not the presence of ketones that causes weight loss, and diets that cause the formation of high levels of ketones are more apt to cause weight gain.

PROTEIN OVERLOAD

I thought that we do not need that much protein. I have been taught that high-protein diets are dangerous. Is that true?

If we define need as the amount necessary to prevent a deficiency disease, then no, we do not need very much protein. As long as you get plenty of fuel, it is hard to become protein deficient. Even if you reduce your food dramatically for several weeks, you will not become protein deficient because your body will break down the muscles for use as a backup source of protein. Sometimes this loss of muscle even causes dramatic numbers of pounds lost on the scale. The drawback about losing muscle is that it hurts your metabolism.

The Metabolism Reset is not a high-protein diet. It is a sufficient-protein diet. The amounts of protein that it provides are good for retaining muscle mass, reducing food cravings, and maintaining metabolic rate. Protein needs become more pronounced when the overall intake of fuel from dietary fat and carbohydrate is lower. This does not mean that the body needs more protein; it just means that it is important to get as much protein as you would on a normal diet despite the reduction of fuel. It takes making protein a priority to achieve this goal, but a healthy metabolism is undoubtedly worth it.

YO-YO DIETING

If I lose weight and then go back to my old habits, is this a yo-yo diet?

No. The average participant loses 9 pounds of fat during each Reset and regains roughly 1 ½ pounds in the following six months. The Maintenance phase does not encourage dieting, but it does encourage habits that lower the risk of weight regain.

Yo-yo diets are good to avoid. They are defined as diets that cause rapid weight loss, mostly from muscle. In these cases, the dieters end up lighter with less metabolic flexibility because they just emptied their glycogen stores. After subsequent cycles of muscle loss and weight regain, they often end up heavier than ever before, with less lean mass as well. Sadly, this places them at risk for all the issues of adiposity: heart disease, diabetes, fatty liver, cancer, brain aging, and early mortality.

When rapid fat loss is done safely, it is a good thing, not a bad thing. In the context of a healthy program, rapid fat loss correlates with greater chances of total fat loss and also greater chances of long-term fat loss. As an example, a study done with diabetics showed that those who lost weight quickest had the greatest odds of becoming nondiabetic. This trend even held true when considering those in the study who regained their weight.[14]

CHRONIC CONDITIONS

THYROID DISEASE

Can I do a Reset if I have a thyroid disease like Hashimoto's or hypothyroidism?

The Metabolism Reset program is safe for those who have thyroid disease. But please do monitor your blood levels before and after embarking on the program, and stay on all treatments as recommended by your health-care provider.

Many people who are on medication to correct their thyroid levels find that they may need less medication after they complete the program. When your liver is reset, your thyroid can function better and your body can better utilize thyroid hormones.

DIABETES

Can I do a Reset if I'm diabetic? What if I'm on meds for my blood sugar?

The Reset program is especially helpful for diabetics. However, it may take close monitoring for those on multiple hypoglycemic medications or insulin. Please talk to your health-care provider and establish a rhythm of daily home checks of your blood sugar. Have your provider give you guidelines to follow in the event that your blood sugar becomes lower than necessary during your Reset.

In our clinic, we have seen hundreds of people who were diabetic and pre-diabetic complete the program and no longer need any medication for diabetes. The danger arises when someone who no longer needs medicine may have her blood sugar levels pushed to dangerously low levels owing to the positive changes brought about by the program. This complication is easy to avoid by working closely with your health-care provider and letting him or her know that you are on a program that may make you need less of your medicine. If you are on medication for diabetes, it is important to check your blood sugar on a daily basis during the Metabolism Reset.

Case Study: Maria

Maria came to us in a state of desperation. At just 33 years old, she was already on medications for her blood pressure, her blood sugar, and her cholesterol levels. Tragically she had seen her mother have a stroke when she was only in her early 50s. It was so severe that she was never able to live independently afterward. Maria was scared to death the same thing would happen to her, because her mother had already been on medications before she had her stroke. Maria had no faith that the medications would protect her, since they didn't protect her mother.

When she first came to see my team, she did not have any prior experience with naturopathic medicine. She was expecting to receive herbs or supplements to take in place of her medications, but was pleasantly surprised when the doctors gave her a diet instead of more pills.

Since we were able to supervise her directly, we had her

stop all her medications on the first day of the Metabolism Reset. Her first blood tests were done two weeks after finishing her first round of the four-week program. For the first time in her life, she had perfect blood tests without medication and her blood pressure was fine. Her blood tests were repeated several times her first year and they all showed the same results—she was doing fine and no longer needed the medications.

DIGESTIVE SYMPTOMS

Can I do the Reset if I have food intolerances?

Yes. The Metabolism Reset already avoids most common food intolerances. If you know that you are sensitive to foods used in certain recipes, exchange those for other foods in the same food category, or with recipes that include foods that you tolerate better. For example, if you are allergic to almonds, feel free to substitute equal quantities of walnuts or other nuts that you do tolerate. If you are allergic to shellfish, try to use other types of seafood or poultry. If you have intolerances, the same rules apply. After the Reset is over, you may choose to test to see if some minor intolerances are still present—assuming your reactions never were severe.

I'm prone to constipation. Will this get worse on the Reset?

Some people notice constipation as a side effect of a reduction in food intake. For those already prone to constipation, it may be even more significant. When you are healthy, you should have a complete bowel movement at least once per day. Also, it should take between about 18 and 24 hours for food to move through the length of your intestinal tract. This is called your bowel's "transit time." You can learn what your transit time is by watching how long after eating beets it takes to see red in your stool, or after taking a few charcoal caps how long it takes your stool to turn black.

If your bowel transit time is longer than 30 hours, it causes more wastes to be reabsorbed into your liver. It also raises the risk for colorectal cancer, although there is some debate as to whether it causes cancer or is associated with cancer.[15] If it is well under 18 hours, it makes it less likely your body can absorb all the essential nutrients from your diet. This can lead to deficiencies in certain nutrients, especially iron, B_{12}, and zinc.

If you notice that during the Reset constipation is more of a problem, here are a few things to try. First, consider your water intake. Are you getting all the recommended glasses each day? Your colon pulls water out of your stool to recycle it for your body's uses. If you are even slightly dehydrated, your colon has to remove so much water from your stool that your stool can be too hard to pass easily. During the Reset, since your food volume is decreased, it is not uncommon for your bowels to have less stool to push through. This should last no longer than the first several days.

The next consideration is fiber intake. Many who are on a diet exclusion that leaves out food categories like legumes, tubers, or intact whole grains may be at risk of getting too little fiber in total, or too few types of fiber overall. If this could be the case, please consider moving to a less restrictive diet, if even just during the Reset.

If constipation is still a problem after taking these steps, you may consider supplemental magnesium. Most people can have regular bowel movements again with as little as a few hundred extra milligrams of magnesium on top of their daily supplementation.

Is the Reset okay to do if I have leaky gut?

The Metabolism Reset will be a great fit for you, just as it is. The diet is high in resistant starch, which is the best-documented food constituent for reversing leaky gut. In fact, studies have shown that resistant starch heals leaky gut through many different mechanisms.

For instance, resistant starch increases bacteroidetes, one of the most important types of good bacteria that people with leaky gut tend to lack. It decreases harmful gram-negative bacteria, and it provides the richest source of butyrate, the main fuel that allows a regrowth of the cells that line the colon.

Some have added butter or ghee (clarified butter) to their diets as an attempt to raise stool butyrate. However, even though these foods contain butyrate, the amounts they contain is insignificant. Butter is typically 3 to 4 percent butyrate by weight.[16] With a teaspoon of butter weighing about 5 grams, this means that it contains roughly 150 mg of butyrate. Studies using oral butyrate found that 8,000 mg was needed to show a clinical change in the colon flora.

Along with resistant starch, the Metabolism Reset is rich in a broad variety of fibers that improve the liver's ability to conjugate wastes. This improvement decreases the flow of harmful substances into the intestinal tract, which harms the flora and causes leaky gut.

I have SIBO (small intestinal bacterial overgrowth) and need to avoid many foods. Can I still do the Reset?

If you are in an active stage of treatment with antibiotics, check with your health-care practitioner to see what is best for you. Many who have been treated for SIBO in the past have found that the Metabolism Reset helps them recover further and become able to tolerate more foods again.

I have candida. Won't eating any carbs make it worse?

The Metabolism Reset avoids processed sugars and is a great approach for someone who has been prone to candida. There has been confusion as to how different foods can affect candida. People who suffer from yeast growth clearly do better when they avoid alcohol and processed sugar; however, carbohydrates are not inherently problematic.

Some authors have recommended that people avoid all foods that contain yeast and foods that are fermented like vinegar and sauerkraut. Yeast overgrowth is a problem of the colon. It can seem intuitive that the foods containing yeast or made from yeast could somehow make this worse. Yet any yeast you swallow would first go through the stomach, where it would be digested long before it would reach the colon.

Even though fermented foods do utilize yeast in their production, they will not cause yeast overgrowth. In fact, most can help it. Vinegar is a powerful topical antifungal—so much so that doctors are trained to prescribe 3 percent acetic acid drops for yeast overgrowth of the ear. And 3 percent acetic acid is the same thing as distilled white vinegar.

Although candida diets should exclude processed sugars, they can make candida worse if they are also too low in healthy carbohydrates like fiber. It is often confusing that chemists use the word *sugar* to refer to any kind of carbohydrate, from Coca-Cola to chickpeas. It is really the processed versions of sugar, such as table sugar and crystalline fructose, that are most important to avoid for those with candida.

PROCESS QUESTIONS

DURATION

Can I stay on the Reset longer than four weeks?

Many people feel so good during the Reset that they wish they could keep going in order to lose more pounds and inches. You can do more Resets, but since we are playing the long game for a better metabolism, I recommend raising your fuel intake for at least two weeks before restarting.

You can do this by adding an extra shake, having a solid lunch, or having one additional meal during the day. Studies have shown that if your fuel intake is low for six weeks or more at a time, you may start to lower your metabolic rate.

The option I recommend for those who are trying to reverse diabetes, high cholesterol, or high blood pressure is to do a Reset once every three months—up to four in the first year. In almost all cases, this is enough to make people no longer need medications or have risks show up on their blood tests.

FUTURE RESETS

Should I Reset in the future, even after hitting my target weight?

Yes, but do not do so more than once annually. Even if you are lean, the Reset process can do a good job ensuring that you stay stable in the coming year. In addition, it yields many benefits apart from fat levels.

These benefits include improving age-related changes to your genes and mitochondria, raising your liver's ability to detoxify environmental wastes, allowing repair of the digestive tract, encouraging the growth of new brain cells, and providing better regulation of hormone levels. Studies on mitochondrial function have shown that protein-sparing modified fasts can give many of the benefits of long-term caloric restriction without the struggle. This process makes mitochondria less damaged by free-radical stress and more able to work in a broader range of fuel availability. This means that you will be more able to keep your weight and energy levels steady despite normal fluctuations in food intake.

The Metabolism Reset can improve your liver function even if you are at a healthy body size. This is important because your liver is essential at protecting you from environmental toxicants and ensuring that your body has a steady supply of vital nutrients necessary for brain and muscle function. It also means your liver will be more able to fine-tune your circulating hormone levels, which will make symptoms of perimenopause and menopause much less significant.

The digestive tract will do especially well with the regular cycle of Resets. The cells that make up the intestinal lining repair themselves every few minutes. Most of the time, this repair cycle is matched by the rate at which cells wear out owing to food digestion. The benefit of a temporary food restriction is that the repair process has time to get ahead of the game.

This cycle also holds true for the portions of the intestinal tract that are secreting digestive fluids, like the stomach and the pancreas. When you give these organs a regular rest, they become more capable of digesting a broader range of foods.

It is especially rewarding to see someone go full circle and regain a state that allows him or her more flexibility in food choices. We all have times when we cannot get the perfect foods we want, owing to social reasons; we eat the same foods as our loved ones are eating. Wouldn't it be great if you could deviate on occasion and not have to pay a price the following days? It is possible to eat well in nearly all cases and have the occasional treat without going off the rails.

Brain cells also benefit from a Reset. In the last decade, one of the most revolutionary findings in all of neurology took place. We now know that adult brain cells can regenerate.

METABOLIC "HACKS"

I've heard that I can boost my metabolism by various hacks, like high-dose green-tea extracts, drinking cold water, or adding cayenne pepper to my meals. Will these help me?

Sorry, but they will not. There are countless hacks, shortcuts, supplements, and weird tricks purported to be revolutionary new shortcuts that promise to raise your metabolism. To be honest, the term "hack" turns me off when applied to health. To me, the word sounds aggressive, violent, and inhumane. Even think of a tool: you can carve, whittle, or fillet with good intent, but no one hacks with good intent. Computers get hacked and we are all the victims. But you cannot hack a garden; you can care for it well or you neglect it.

The idea that you can trick a living thing into producing some particular outcome ignores the fact that we are systems with mind-boggling degrees of internal regulation, most of which are oblivious to us. Most hacks, if they do anything, end up with the body's resisting the change and doing the opposite. The other problem is that even if we could hack a certain result in the short term, who knows what it will do decades down the road? End of rant.

This said, most hacks rely on the effects of cold or on supplements that either act as stimulants or prevent you from absorbing calories. First, for the cold: Yes, it is true. If you drink 16 ounces of ice water on an empty stomach, your body does expend calories in the process of heating the water to room temperature. To be specific, it burns about 8 calories, which would allow you to enjoy 9 extra blueberries.[17]

Cold has been used in many other ways, such as ice-water baths and spending time in colder weather. Being in cold does make your body work harder to stay warmer, but it also raises the appetite and stimulates subcutaneous fat growth. Arctic mammals like whales, seals, and polar bears are not known for being svelte. I grew up in northern Minnesota. Each winter day's national weather report said that my hometown was either the coldest spot in the country or just a few miles from it. If cold worked the way people make it out, we all should have been bikini models by spring. We were not.

Stimulants like coffee, tea, ephedra, and yerba mate do raise your metabolic rate by a few percent, but they also increase the alpha 2 receptors on your adipose cells. This means that your fat cells cut in line in front of your muscle cells when your bloodstream is passing out fuel. Absorption blockers make your intestinal tract absorb less fat or less carbohydrate. Neither blocks more than a few percentages of what you eat, but all can cause malabsorption of nutrients and fecal incontinence—aka unplanned #2. They also tend to raise your appetite by twice as many calories as they block. For every 20 calories they block, you will end up eating 40 calories more.

chapter eleven

Troubleshooting

FOOD CRAVINGS

How do you get through the Metabolism Reset if you feel hungry all the time and your cravings are out of control? It can seem like food cravings are completely overwhelming and impossible to resist. Yet those that come on intensely are always due to biochemical reasons. Once you figure out the reason, you can regain your freedom.

Reset your taste buds. If you crave certain tastes, your taste buds may be to blame. Processed and ultra-processed foods like flour products, juices, and snack foods can make your palate numb to the tastes found in unprocessed foods. Even when you eat enough to satisfy you, your tongue does not register the tastes well enough to help turn off hunger.

Your taste buds work via receptors. If you taste something that is sick-eningly sweet often enough, some of your sweet receptors shut off. You will no longer be able to appreciate subtle sweet flavors. The same is true for salty foods. For example, if you ate nothing but pure white sugar, your taste buds would become so numbed to the sweet taste that sweet fruits like mango would taste sour or bitter to you. This exact thing happened to a woman who was on my friend JJ Virgin's show called *Freaky Eaters*. It was challenging for her to eat anything besides pure sugar, but over the course of a week avoiding it completely, she developed more normal taste buds.

The more you limit your exposure to powerful tastes like sweet and salty, the more receptors your taste buds grow and the more you appreciate the taste even when it is subtle. By focusing on the minimally processed foods in the Metabolism Reset, you will soon find that oats, potatoes, lentils, and whole fruits satisfy your sweet taste. You will also find that vegetables, mushrooms, and seafood naturally have enough salty and savory flavors as they are, without much if any seasoning.

Over time, the taste buds do recalibrate themselves, but thankfully there are some ways to speed the process. Here are a couple of options based on which foods you crave the most.

IF YOU CRAVE SWEETS

Avoid all sweet-tasting things for 48 hours. Even safe sweeteners such as stevia and xylitol may be culprits for some people. Avoid concentrated sweet flavors like diet sodas and chewing gum. Also, do not use sweeteners and flavors in your shakes or beverages during this stage.

Other sources of sugar and sweet taste that can inadvertently work their way into the Reset include fruit and sweetened milk substitutes that some people mistakenly add to their shake. If you are trying to reset your sweet taste buds, consider the original Reset Shake (see page 119) and try making it with only water.

Here is the nuclear option for sugar cravings. There is an Ayurvedic herb called gurmar, which means the "destroyer of sugar." Its Latin name is *Gymnema sylvestre*. If you hold it in contact with your tongue for a minute, your sweet taste buds completely turn off. It is a harmless albeit bizarre experience that lasts for a few hours. You can use gurmar in a couple ways. One is to do a switch with it several times per day on a schedule. The other is to use it to make you averse to some food that seems to take control over you. While your sweet taste buds are numb, go ahead and indulge in the very food you crave. Go ahead, try it. We had some at home one time and my daughter wanted to see how it would affect her craving for caramel candies. Years later, she still cannot stand the thought of them. What happens is that the food has almost no flavor; it seems like you are eating dirt or cardboard.

Here is how to do it. Buy either capsules or the powdered form of the plant. Mix either $1/2$ teaspoon of the powder or the powder from five 500 mg capsules stirred into $1/2$ cup water. Gargle the water in your mouth for two minutes, then spit it out. You can repeat as needed to combat sweet cravings, but most find that a few treatments are all that they need.

IF YOU CRAVE SALTY FOODS

It is possible to follow the guidelines of the Metabolism Reset while still being on a high-salt diet if you add too much salt in your cooking or at the table. Thankfully, salt tastes often can be adjusted faster than sweet tastes. The less salt you use, the less you will crave. For the first one or two days, your food will taste bland and flavorless, but soon you will notice the shift and even the smallest amount of salt will be too much for you.

To speed the process, you can add potassium chloride to your food after cooking. Table salt is sodium chloride, and it is likely that the cravings and harmful effects in excess are more related to the sodium than to the chloride. Potassium chloride lacks this baggage and will still let your taste receptors reset. Most grocery stores carry this as the U.S. products NuSalt or LiteSalt.

Savory-tasting foods can also reduce salt cravings, as well as cravings in general. Savory tastes, also called umami, are controlled by a taste receptor that has a two-phase effect on appetite. In the first phase, savory foods increase the enjoyment of the meal. This response is helpful because you'll find yourself more satisfied by simple, minimally processed foods. You will feel less of a drive for foods that are sugary, salty, or high in fat. In the second phase, savory foods make you feel full longer and you won't need as much food. They leave you feeling more satisfied, causing you to eat less afterward.

One of the strongest versions of umami is the synthetic flavor enhancer monosodium glutamate. Thankfully, many natural foods contain safe and natural forms of glutamate that give the same umami benefit without the concerns associated with monosodium glutamate. Good examples of these include sun-dried tomatoes, shiitake mushrooms, Thai or Vietnamese fish sauce, potatoes, nutritional yeast, green tea, and tamari, or wheat-free soy sauce.

Sun-dried tomatoes, especially those not packed in oil, are easy to dice and add to nearly any vegetable dish. Dried shiitake mushrooms are one of my favorite pantry staples. They are inexpensive and have an indefinite shelf life. And along with the umami taste, shiitake mushrooms are also excellent immune tonics and adaptogens. You can soak the dried mushrooms in warm water for 20 minutes, and use them like fresh button mushrooms in any dish. You can also break them up into small pieces and drop them into legumes or grains while you are cooking them.

A final great trick is to grind shiitake mushrooms into a powder using a blender or a coffee grinder. Add several teaspoons of this powder and some water in the final phases of sautéing any mixture of vegetables. You will end up with the delicate and savory gravy reminiscent of the ubiquitous canned cream of mushroom soup used in so many less healthy recipes.

Green tea in cooking? Yes, one of the easiest applications is to add three bags of green tea to 1 quart of water, simmer for two minutes, and use to poach fish or poultry.

Nutritional yeast is another great natural flavor enhancer. Along with the flavor, it also provides quality protein and many B vitamins and minerals, including zinc and selenium. One consideration is to find nutritional yeast that is not fortified with synthetic B vitamins. Most brands are, and the big problem is that they contain synthetic folic acid, which can raise the risk for certain cancers in many people with common genetic variations.

Nutritional yeast has a flavor similar to Parmesan cheese. I like to add about a teaspoon to a stir-fry near the end of cooking. Start with small amounts, as it is easy to get too much and overpower the taste of the dish.

FAT CRAVINGS

Many low-carb enthusiasts have found that they have a "fat tooth" that is hard to shake. The same ideas apply—you'll miss it less after eating less. One of the easiest ways to reduce cravings for fat is the ancient practice of tongue scraping. Ayurvedic medicine has recommended this practice for thousands of years in order to improve overall health and digestion.

Modern science tells us that the service of the tongue contracts bacteria in food residue and holds on to them for days. Many people brush their tongue; however, this mostly just moves about such food particles and does not remove residue the way scraping can.

Look for a tongue scraper online or from larger health food stores. These scrapers are made of porcelain, steel, or plastic. Avoid plastic, but porcelain or steel is fine, although porcelain can break over time. The scrapers are shaped like a letter U. You hold the ends between each thumb and forefinger, reach the band to the back of your tongue, and gently scrape it across the top of your tongue, moving forward. Repeat once or twice or until the whitish material is no longer visible on the scraper.

Along with reducing your craving for fat, this may also reduce your craving for sweet foods, give you better breath, and improve your digestion. This practice can also prevent the loss of taste sensitivity that many develop with age.

NO WEIGHT LOSS

Help! You are doing everything right, yet the inches are not budging. What gives? Please read through all these scenarios before you assume one cannot apply to you. Some of these pitfalls are really counterintuitive, and I have been surprised how much better someone can do after changing something that may not at first have seemed like all that big a deal.

Many such habits seem like they could not possibly be relevant, because they have been part of your life for years. Yet this is a case where a seemingly harmless bystander could be a hidden culprit. That one thing you did on a daily basis that you thought didn't matter could be that one thing that has been holding back your progress. Even if you think one of these habits does not apply to you, try addressing it anyway and see what happens. If nothing changes, you'll know for sure. If things suddenly get better, you'll gain more control over your health.

CHECK YOUR GLANDS

THYROID

Of all the medical issues that make weight loss harder, none succeeds nearly as well as thyroid disease. Current estimates are that thyroid disease affects as many as 25 percent of American adults. Of these, only about 5 percent have been identified and are on treatment, but only about 2.5 percent have had their symptoms controlled by treatment.

Healing your thyroid could be an important part of keeping your metabolism healthy, even if you've never suspected thyroid disease, or you are already on treatment for thyroid disease, or even if you have been told you do not have thyroid disease. Thyroid disease is more common among adult women, and it often comes on after pregnancy or around menopause. Along with a slow metabolism, it can cause fatigue, hair loss, muscle pain, dry skin, and digestive symptoms—although rarely all at once. Most people with thyroid disease have only two or three of the symptoms. It is more suspicious when the symptoms come on over an apparent timeframe, as opposed to symptoms that have been present all along to varying degrees.

Thyroid hormones directly control how much fuel the body turns into energy and how much fuel the body sends to storage. This is the reason why so many people with thyroid disease have a combination of easy weight gain and fatigue. Too much fuel is stored, leading to fat retention, and little fuel is burned, leading to fatigue. The good news is that thyroid disease is treatable. For many, it's possible to restore the thyroid to normal function. For nearly all, the thyroid symptoms can be reversed with safe and natural treatment.

Many years ago, I created a free quiz that can help you see whether your thyroid is responsible for any of your ongoing symptoms. You can find it at thethyroidquiz.com. Even if you have never suspected thyroid disease, or think you are already on effective treatment for it, it is worth taking the quiz. If your score is elevated, the quiz will give you suggestions on how to find a good doctor to work with and what you should expect to do in order to help your thyroid so that you can feel better.

Case Study: Margaret

Margaret was a 44-year-old woman who came to see me about her thyroid. She had been on treatment with Synthroid for over five years and she never lost the weight she first put on when her thyroid slowed down about six years ago. First, I guided Margaret through a change in medication and treatment of several of the causes of her autoimmunity. These changes helped her fatigue and her hair loss, and they also helped her lose about 12 of the extra 20 pounds she had been carrying.

Although I recommended the Reset at first, Margaret wanted to see how much would happen with thyroid treatment alone. Once her thyroid levels had stabilized, she agreed to go on the four-week Reset. By the end of the four weeks, she was amazed that she had lost another 9 pounds and was now actually 1 pound lighter than her goal weight.

Immediately after the Reset, I asked Margaret to recheck her thyroid levels because in many cases, people need less thyroid medication either because their bodies are so much lighter or because their own thyroid function has improved. The change in Margaret's thyroid levels was dramatic. She needed several reductions in her dose and in the months following the diet, she was able to stay on about half as much thyroid medicine as she needed before.

How is this possible? The triglycerides trapped inside the liver can have harmful effects on the immune system and even can trigger autoimmunity. In Margaret's case, it seemed they were one of the main triggers for her autoimmune thyroid disease.

ADRENALS

The adrenal glands make a hormone called cortisol, which controls where fuel is sent in the body. Cortisol is made in a distinct rhythm throughout the day, called the cortisol slope. Healthy people make the day's highest amount of cortisol when they wake up and then they stop making cortisol as they wind down and prepare for sleep.

With chronic stress, this cortisol slope can become altered in three main ways that move across a spectrum from mildest to most significant. In the mildest form, "Stressed," the high levels of morning cortisol persist throughout the night. In the middle form, "Wired and Tired," the morning cortisol becomes low while the nighttime levels become high—opposite the ideal cortisol slope. In the most severe form, "Crashed," cortisol never elevates in the morning and it stays low all throughout the day. To date, thousands of studies have shown that this cortisol slope is a significant predictor of fat retention, physical disease, mental illness, and early death. In fact, in the Whitehall II study, it was shown that nonsmokers with an abnormal cortisol slope were more susceptible to early death than were smokers within normal cortisol slope. It was also a stronger predictor of early death than was cholesterol, blood sugar, body weight, or blood pressure. Yes, it is a big deal.

In the late 1990s, many alternative practitioners called this phenomenon "adrenal fatigue" and claimed that it resulted from a weakness of the adrenal glands from overwork. However, in the case of an abnormal cortisol slope, it is not that the adrenal glands are unable to make cortisol. Rather, the hypothalamic–pituitary axis is intentionally slowing down the cortisol production so that the body has a chance to rest and repair.

Adrenal-fatigue advocates were correct in identifying many symptoms of an abnormal cortisol slope and in identifying many factors of diet and lifestyle that can contribute to its becoming abnormal. Because the term "adrenal fatigue" implies a situation that is not the case, most conventional doctors and endocrinologists do not consider this a valid diagnosis. However, the problems of an abnormal cortisol slope and their effects upon fat retention are all too real.

When your cortisol levels are healthy, more fuel is sent to your muscle tissue. When cortisol levels are unhealthy, the body can more readily go into fight-or-flight mode. This fight-or-flight response also has another "f" that goes with it—famine. Chronic stress signals food scarcity. Your body is more careful to store fuel as visceral fat and becomes reluctant to burn fuel that it may not need to. In fact, in a chronic stress state, visceral fat also makes more cortisol, leading to a vicious cycle.

An abnormal cortisol slope can cause many symptoms, such as general fatigue, insomnia, anxiety, muscle cramps, and dizziness. Anyone who has these symptoms should suspect cortisol slope abnormalities. Because the adrenal glands change their function throughout the day, one can especially suspect adrenal abnormalities with symptoms that predictably get better or worse at predictable times each day. Say, each afternoon you become exhausted and feel the need for coffee or sugar. Or, say, that early each morning around 2 or 3 o'clock you wake up and your mind is racing. The specific timing of both of those symptoms makes it more likely that they are caused by the adrenals.

Because your adrenal glands help control your blood sugar levels, they can be involved with many symptoms of hypoglycemia, such as fatigue or mood changes before meals, as well as a craving for sugar. Because the adrenal glands also control blood electrolyte levels, they can also trigger symptoms of salt craving, dizziness when standing suddenly, or nighttime leg cramps.

What to do if you suspect abnormal adrenal function: There are abnormalities of cortisol slope and there are overt adrenal diseases, such as Addison's disease and Cushing's syndrome. Most doctors and endocrinologists are able to identify adrenal diseases, but most cannot identify abnormalities of cortisol slope. If you suspect that your adrenal glands are not working right, it is best to test for both adrenal disease and cortisol slope abnormalities.

Blood tests are good for the first round of testing when it comes to evaluating adrenal diseases. Salivary (spit) tests are better for identifying cortisol slope abnormalities because they allow you to see how cortisol changes across the course of the day. A blood test cannot do this as well typically because they are only done once and because the stress of having a blood test done can skew cortisol levels.

Even without seeing a doctor, you can get a good sense of how likely you are to have cortisol slope abnormalities with a simple survey of your symptoms. First, take one week to write down any unusual symptoms you notice, how severe they are, and how often you notice them. Once you have them, take the free survey at adrenalquiz.com. I compiled results of many cortisol slope tests along with symptoms described by hundreds of people, and was able to find out which symptoms best predicted which of the cortisol slope abnormalities. By taking the quiz, you will learn how likely it is that your adrenals are causing your symptoms, and if so exactly which level they are at right now.

What to do if you have an abnormal cortisol slope: Cortisol abnormalities can heal. Even the worst really take no more than several months to return to optimal. There are many strategies to help with that including relaxation exercises, herbal medicines, acupuncture, and stress reduction. My top three recommendations are carb cycling, light therapies, and journaling.

Carb cycling works because healthy carbohydrates can lower cortisol. If your diet is too low in carbohydrates, your body makes more cortisol to convert your muscle tissue into blood sugar. Remember that a healthy cortisol slope involves the lowest cortisol levels in the evening. Because of that, the evening is a good time to have some healthy carbohydrates. The ones that work best to lower cortisol are the same ones used in the Metabolism Reset: potatoes, legumes, vegetable starches like squash, and intact whole grains like buckwheat. Carb cycling is the main concept behind the success of the Adrenal Reset Diet. In a clinical trial, this approach was shown to improve the cortisol slope by over 50 percent within 30 days.

Light therapies work because natural sunlight in the morning is the main queue that sets your cortisol cycle for the whole day. Even though we always turn on the lights to get ready in the morning, indoor light is not bright enough nor is it the same wavelength as sunlight. Read more about light therapies in the section about insomnia in Chapter 6.

Journaling is a powerful habit that can improve the cortisol slope, as well as your entire stress response. It works because the act of forming feelings into words moves the feelings out of parts of the brain in which they stay stuck and into parts of the brain that allow them to resolve. An effective habit is to take five minutes each evening and write down any random thoughts that come to mind. When we think thoughts, we may not resolve them or dissipate the emotional sway they hold over us. But when we form them into language, they lose their charge and we decrease our chronic levels of stress. The fascinating part is that it does not seem to matter whether or not anyone hears or reads our words, just that we form them.

LIMIT THE UNLIMITED?

What exactly does "unlimited" mean? To most people, in most cases, it means just that. However, if you have had large quantities of unlimited foods and have seen no progress, you may be sensitive to food volume.

This is a rare problem, but I have had people tell me that they got in the habit of eating quarts of unlimited food throughout the day. At some point, the small amount of fuel from the unlimited foods can add up. There is also a phenomenon by which if you stretch your stomach too much you can activate alpha receptors that cause your liver to dump glucose into your bloodstream.

If this could be you, limit your unlimited foods—as paradoxical as that sounds. See if it helps to keep each snack under 2 cups of food volume.

DETOX SYMPTOMS

Don't ignore your symptoms. You could have some medical mishap occur that has nothing to do with your Reset, so do not ignore it. Some detox symptoms can happen, but when in doubt, see your health-care provider.

During the first few days, you can expect some symptoms to show up as your liver is resetting itself. These can include food cravings, mild headaches, poor quality sleep, mood changes, fatigue, and in some cases muscle aches. Please do not be alarmed by these symptoms if they do show up. Know that they will not last and welcome them as signs of progress. They happen because your liver is clearing out trapped triglycerides that made it unable to function. The worse you feel during detox, the more you needed it and the better you will do afterward. For most people, these detox symptoms diminish greatly starting on the third day and are usually no longer significant by the time the first week is over.

The point is, plan for them to occur, and if possible arrange for your first few days to take place during times when they will not be as significant. For example, do not plan for your first two days to take place at the beginning of a long-awaited trip or on the day you have to give a big presentation.

GAS AND BLOATING

The Metabolism Reset provides an average of over 40 grams of fiber per day from a broad range of fiber categories. These fibers are an important part of helping the liver work better, improve blood sugar, and reduce food cravings. People who begin the program after doing the popular paleo or low-carb diets often have not eaten legumes, potatoes, or intact whole grains for some time. Such a restrictive diet can lead to a lack of diversity in the bowel flora. Thankfully, the bowel flora can quickly rebound with the introduction of a broader variety of healthy fiber-rich foods. However, sometimes this improvement in the flora comes at the cost of some initial adjustment symptoms. This happens because dormant species of flora are giving off methane and other by-products. This extra gas can cause bloating and other associated symptoms.

How do you make the Reset easier? Well, how do you like to take off a Band-Aid? If you like to do it fast and be done with it, do nothing; these symptoms will go away on their own, typically in three to ten days. If you prefer to take off a Band-Aid slowly, then simply introduce fiber-rich foods more gradually, especially legumes.

Legumes are often the food category with some of the largest benefits and therefore the largest tendency to cause symptoms when you're not used to them. Many people make the mistake of thinking they are somehow intolerant or unable to digest legumes, which likely isn't true. Try adding a single tablespoon of pinto beans to your diet each day for two weeks. This is so little that almost no one experiences any symptoms or side effects from the addition. By then, you should be able to begin eating beans in just about any quantity and frequency.

FOOD INTOLERANCES

The main culprit behind new digestive symptoms when there's a change in diet is food intolerances. These come in two main types: immediate-onset and delayed. You can find many debates about whether intolerances should be categorized as allergies, sensitivities, or reactions. The differences in these labels may be relevant to doctors or researchers, but they aren't relevant to a person who is miserable.

The immediate-onset reactions are the most apparent and typically are figured out at earlier stages in life. These reactions cause dramatic symptoms like rashes, difficulty breathing, or swelling of the body. They are driven by IgE antibodies, which are found in the gut and in the skin, which is why they can be detected by skin tests. These reactions are also the least apt to change over time. Most people who have had any always will have them and they have been aware of them for quite some time.

Some foods are more prone to become immediate intolerances than others. Most common culprits include peanuts, shellfish, strawberries, onions, and soy products. If you suspect an immediate reaction, avoid the food completely until you can work with the doctor and come to an understanding of the symptoms. Even if these reactions seemed mild, it is possible that they can become severe and even life-threatening with repeated exposure.

The other main category of food reactions is that of delayed intolerances. These reactions can take as long as days or weeks to cause symptoms, and the symptoms are often more vague and nebulous. Common symptoms of delayed reactions include bloating, headaches, joint pain, irritability, brain fog, and fatigue. Some of the most common food culprits include wheat, dairy, eggs, almonds, and cranberries. Unlike immediate reactions, these types of delayed reactions can change over time. It is common that people develop these even if they did not have them in the past, but they can also improve as digestive function gets better.

These delayed intolerances are driven by various antibodies, including IgG, IgA, and IgD. Because these are often not found on the skin, skin tests do not predict these reactions. Because they take a while to show up, even blood tests can be inconsistent at showing them.

Celiac disease is an example of a delayed intolerance driven by IgA antibodies. Like other types, blood tests may fail to identify it. Unlike other delayed intolerances, though, it is unlikely to improve over time.

Most of these food culprits are foods that have long, complex protein chains. When these protein chains are not well digested, they can circulate and trigger a gradual immune response. It can also happen that people feel reactions to foods simply because they have not eaten that food often in the recent past.

As important as it is to avoid processed junk food, it is also important to eat as large a diversity of natural foods as possible. Many popular diets are based on avoiding entire categories of foods such as legumes, nuts, seafood, dairy, whole grains, and fruits and vegetables high in phytonutrients. Such food restrictions inevitably lead to risks of nutrient deficiency and a "lazy" digestive tract.

Case Study: Danielle

Danielle wanted to try the Metabolism Reset after reading some of my blog posts. She was 49 at the time and had an extra 25 pounds that seemed to show up out of the blue when she started perimenopause. She had read testimonials about typical results and thought that it all sounded perfect. Although she first had a goal of weight loss, she realized that the inches were more important. She thought it would be great if she could lose about 4 inches from around her waist.

Unfortunately, she barely lost half an inch on her first Reset. She talked to people in the support group on my site and realized what went wrong. One was that she used a whey-based protein in her shakes. Whey protein can contain bovine sources of growth hormones such as IGF-1 in levels that can be higher than those found in other dairy foods. These growth hormones may be useful for athletes seeking muscle growth, but they can make it hard for women who are trying to lose inches.

Danielle also realized that she was taking supplements that contained extra iodine, which could slow her thyroid function. After a one-month hiatus, she attempted the Reset again, this time with an iodine-free multivitamin and the original Reset Shake (see page 119) used in the clinical trial.

The second time at Reset worked like a charm! She dropped over 3 $\frac{1}{2}$ inches in no time and was doubly pleased to no longer need a restrictive diet. Now she eats intuitively and stays trim.

FATIGUE

What if you feel unusually tired after the first week of the program? This can happen for reasons that can fall into two big categories: (1) some underlying cause of fatigue has become more apparent, or (2) you are not doing some part of the program.

There are many causes of fatigue and if you experienced fatigue before, it is normal for it to be worse when you are on a low-fuel diet. Here are some of the top causes to consider.

HYPOGLYCEMIA

If you notice that your symptoms are worse before your meal or shake and improve afterward, then you may have hypoglycemia. The easiest work-around is to get as much resistant starch as possible and to make sure you are getting each recommended serving of protein. Each time you eat a meal high in resistant starch, you have the opportunity to stabilize your blood sugar for the following seven to nine hours. These beneficial effects linger to a lesser degree for a full 24 hours. The steadier your blood sugar levels are, the steadier your energy levels will be.

IRON DEFICIENCY

During the Reset, your diet may contain less iron, since it is high in plant proteins. It is also higher in fibers, which can bind some iron from the diet. If you have an untreated iron deficiency, this combination can leave you more tired. You can suspect this if you also notice headaches, are prone to hair loss, and your symptoms are worse during your menstrual cycle.

If you suspect an iron deficiency, talk to your health-care provider, get tested for anemia, and follow the recommended treatment. Please also be sure to retest after three months to confirm you are getting better. In many cases, people are given supplements of a type or dosage that may not be effective for them.

MICRONUTRIENTS

Fatigue can come from a lack of nearly any micronutrient. Because your diet is limited during the Reset, the multivitamin becomes more significant. Please revisit Chapter 6 and review the discussions on how to select a multivitamin.

OVERACTIVITY

If you are really tired, it is possible that nothing is wrong but you are just overdoing it. Along with reducing your exercise, your Reset can work better when you are not taking on a dozen projects. Stress and prolonged intense mental activity do take their toll on the body, making it more difficult to be intentional about your food choices and your food quantities. Instead, think of this time as extending to more than just your food. When you slow down on your own terms, you will come back stronger than ever.

WHAT IF WEIGHT LOSS IS TOO FAST?

Even though "waist loss" is the ultimate goal of the program, some people are surprised by how fast their weight drops. If your waist-to-height ratio was well over 0.5 before the Reset, it may not be uncommon to see a weight change of up to 10 pounds in the first week and as much as 20 pounds in the first month. As always, please check with your health-care provider for anything that seems unusual for you.

If your weight-loss rate is higher than this or seems alarming, here are a few things to think about.

FOOD PORTIONS

Are you consuming the full amount of protein in your shakes? Many popular protein powders have less than the recommended amounts, so please double-check the label. If your protein intake is lower than recommended, you might lose too much muscle mass. Those who avoid certain categories of protein may also find themselves falling behind on the recommended protein intake of their meals. Even though this can cause more pounds to come off at first, it will just set you up for more problems with your metabolism in the future.

Are you getting all the recommended parts of your meal, including the carbohydrates? Many people attempt to consume less food than recommended with the hope of achieving quicker results. In both these cases, even if scale weight loss seems to be fast, it is important to remember that the real goal is long-term waist loss and that long-term success hinges on how well you retain your muscle tissue.

STILL LOSING TOO FAST

If you are doing all the right things, and you are still dropping pounds faster than you wish, you can continue your Reset and still get the benefits by changing from (a) two shakes, one meal, and unlimited snacks (2-1-∞) to (b) two shakes, two meals, and unlimited snacks (2-2-∞). There are a certain number of people who find this second option more effective. Many of these people are men used to high amounts of exercise, or just larger-sized people in general.

HOW TO MAINTAIN WITH
HIGH LEVELS OF EXERCISE

Remember that the Reset will be most effective if you reduce exercise to the recommended amounts in Chapter 6. However, this may not be possible for those of you who do hard physical work. In these cases, follow the program as recommended, but add one extra meal for every two hours per day spent on physical work and every one hour per day spent in exercise. Do know that you still may see short-term fat-loss benefits from this approach, but you may not see the lasting changes in your metabolism.

If you are an athlete, schedule your Reset to coincide with the earliest stages of your recovery season. There is just no way you will benefit from the Reset if you are burning high amounts of fuel on a daily basis.

Great job on getting through the book! I hope the program worked as well for you as it has for others.

Now what? If this book allowed you to retire from a career of professional dieting, what does retirement look like? Well, you probably know a lot about this stuff by now. I'm pretty sure this was not the first book you've read on food and nutrition. It would be sad to take a whole bunch of experience and knowledge and not put it to good use.

At the end of the day, the best use we can make of our time is to make things a little better for someone else. Consider yourself deputized to share some of the insights you've learned from this book. Food is not the enemy. Carbs are not evil. Beating yourself up is not the answer.

Do what you can to model what works for the younger generation. I feel like each coming generation is getting more vulnerable to being trapped in fads and health is no exception.

If you have considered a career in health, there is no better time to start. There are many excellent training programs for health coaches and nutritionists. A few favorites of mine are the Functional Nutrition Alliance and the Institute for Transformative Nutrition.

Please know that you are not in this by yourself. I always love hearing from you. If you have any feedback, it would mean the world to me if you would share it. Please tell me any insights you had, how the experience went, and any ways you found to make it work even better for you. You can always connect with me at drc@drchristianson.com. I read every email and personally reply to many of them.

To your health,
Dr. Alan Christianson

INTRODUCTION

1   "The State of Childhood Obesity." The State of Childhood Obesity—The State of Obesity. Accessed December 16, 2017. https://stateofobesity.org/childhood -obesity-trends/.

CHAPTER TWO: YOUR LIVER HOLDS THE KEY

1   Taub, Rebecca. "Liver Regeneration: From Myth to Mechanism." *Nature Reviews Molecular Cell Biology* 5, no. 10 (2004): 836–47. doi:10.1038/nrm1489.

2   https://www.ncbi.nlm.nih.gov/pubmedhealth/PMH0072577/.

3   Ibid.

4   "Metabolic Functions of the Liver." http://www.vivo.colostate.edu/hbooks /pathphys/digestion/liver/metabolic.html.

5   Ones, E. A. "Milestones in Research on Hepatic Encephalopathy." *Hepatic Encephalopathy and Nitrogen Metabolism.* 2017;6:1637. 555–72. doi:10.1007/1-4020-4456-9_46.

6   Aizawa, Toru, Takashi Yamada, Masato Tawata, Takuo Shimizu, Seiichi Furuta, Kendo Kiyosawa, and Minoru Yakata. "Thyroid Hormone Metabolism

in Patients with Liver Cirrhosis, as Judged by Urinary Excretion of Triiodo-thyronine." *Journal of the American Geriatrics Society* 28, no. 11 (1980): 485–91. doi:10.1111/j.1532-5415.1980.tb01126.x.

7   Huang, Miau-Ju, and Yun-Fan Liaw. "Clinical Associations Between Thyroid And Liver Diseases." *Journal of Gastroenterology and Hepatology* 10, no. 3 (1995): 344–50. doi:10.1111/j.1440-1746.1995.tb01106.x.

8   Stewart, P. M. "11 Beta-Hydroxysteroid Dehydrogenase Deficiency and Glu-cocorticoid Status in Patients with Alcoholic and Non-Alcoholic Chronic Liver Disease." *Journal of Clinical Endocrinology & Metabolism* 76, no. 3 (1993): 748–51. doi:10.1210/jc.76.3.748.

9   Asensio, C., P. Muzzin, and F. Rohner-Jeanrenaud. "Role of Glucocorticoids in the Physiopathology of Excessive Fat Deposition and Insulin Resistance." *International Journal of Obesity* 28, no. S4 (2004). S45 – 52. doi:10.1038/sj.ijo.0802856.

10   Jirillo, E., D. Caccavo, T. Magrone, E. Piccigallo, L. Amati, A. Lembo, C. Kalis, and M. Gumenscheimer. "The Role of the Liver in the Response to LPS: Experimental and Clinical Findings." *Journal of Endotoxin Research* 8, no. 5 (2002): 319–27. doi:10.1179/096805102125000641.

11   Bilzer, Manfred, Frigga Roggel, and Alexander L. Gerbes. "Role of Kuep-fer Cells in Host Defense and Liver Disease." *Liver International* 26, no. 10 (2006): 1175–86. doi:10.1111/j.1478-3231.2006.01342.x.

12   Rachek, Lyudmila I. "Free Fatty Acids and Skeletal Muscle Insulin Resis-tance." *Progress in Molecular Biology and Translational Science Glucose Homeostatis and the Pathogenesis of Diabetes Mellitus*, no. 121 (2014): 267–92. doi:10.1016/b978-0-12-800101-1.00008-9.

13   Richter, Erik A., Bente Sonne, Kari J. Mikines, Thorkil Ploug, and Henrik Galbo. "Muscle and Liver Glycogen, Protein, and Triglyceride in the Rat." *European Journal of Applied Physiology and Occupational Physiology* 52, no. 3 (1984): 346–50. doi:10.1007/bf01015225.

14   Huang, Tao, Yan Zheng, Adela Hruby, Donald A. Williamson, George A. Bray, Yiru Shen, Frank M. Sacks, and Lu Qi. "Dietary Protein Modifies the Effect of the MC4R Genotype on 2-Year Changes in Appetite and Food Crav-ing: The POUNDS Lost Trial." *Journal of Nutrition*, no. 147 (3) (2017): 439-444. doi:10.3945/jn.116.242958.\

15   Papakonstantinou, E., D. Triantafillidou, D. B. Panagiotakos, A. Koutso-vasilis, M. Saliaris, A. Manolis, A. Melidonis, and A. Zampelas. "A High-Protein Low-Fat Diet Is More Effective in Improving Blood Pressure and Triglycerides in Calorie-Restricted Obese Individuals With Newly Diagnosed Type 2 Diabetes." *European Journal of Clinical Nutrition* 64, no. 6 (2010): 595–602. doi:10.1038/ejcn.2010.29.

16   Schiavo, Luigi, Giuseppe Scalera, Vincenzo Pilone, Gabriele De Sena, Vin-cenzo Quagliariello, Antonio Iannelli, and Alfonso Barbarisi. "A Comparative Study Examining the Impact of a Protein-Enriched Vs Normal Protein Post-operative Diet on Body Composition and Resting Metabolic Rate in Obese Patients after Sleeve Gastrectomy." *Obesity Surgery* 27, no. 4 (2016): 881–88. doi:10.1007/s11695-016-2382-y.

17   Newman, John C., and Eric Verdin. "β-Hydroxybutyrate: A Signaling Me-
      tabolite." *Annual Review of Nutrition* 37, no. 1 (2017): 51–76. doi:10.1146/
      annurev-nutr-071816-064916.

18   Hall, Kevin D., Kong Y. Chen, Juen Guo, Yan Y. Lam, Rudolph L. Leibel,
      Laurel Es Mayer, Marc L. Reitman, Michael Rosenbaum, Steven R. Smith,
      B. Timothy Walsh, and Eric Ravussin. "Energy Expenditure and Body
      Composition Changes After an Isocaloric Ketogenic Diet in Overweight and
      Obese Men." *American Journal of Clinical Nutrition* 104, no. 2 (2016): 324–33.
      doi:10.3945/ajcn.116.133561.

19   "Protect Your Family from Exposures to Lead." EPA. August 30, 2017. https://
      www.epa.gov/lead/protect-your-family-exposures-lead.

20   "Toxic Substances Portal - Chloroform." Centers for Disease Control and
      Prevention. January 21, 2015. https://www.atsdr.cdc.gov/phs/phs.asp?id=51
      &tid=16.

21   "Is Butter Back?" Dr. Alan Christianson. http://drchristianson.com/is-butter
      -back/.

22   "Tox Town—Polyvinyl Chloride (PVC)—Toxic chemicals and environmental
      health risks where you live and work—Text Version." U.S. National Library
      of Medicine. 2017. https://toxtown.nlm.nih.gov/text_version/chemicals.php
      ?id=84.

23   Wahlang, Banrida, Juliane I. Beier, Heather B. Clair, Heather J. Bellis-
      Jones, K. Cameron Falkner, Craig J. Mcclain, and Matt C. Cave. "Toxicant-
      associated Steatohepatitis." *Toxicologic Pathology* 41, no. 2 (2012): 343–60.
      doi:10.1177/0192623312468517.

24   Roberts, Michael S., Beatrice M. Magnusson, Frank J. Burczynski, and Mi-
      chael Weiss. "Enterohepatic Circulation." *Clinical Pharmacokinetics* 41, no. 10
      (2002): 751–90. doi:10.2165/00003088-200241100-00005.

25   Karandish, Majid, Mahtab Tamimi, Ali Akbar Shayesteh, Mohammad
      Hosein Haghighizadeh, and Mohammad Taha Jalali. "The Effect of Mag-
      nesium Supplementation and Weight Loss on Liver Enzymes in Patients
      With Nonalcoholic Fatty Liver Disease." *Journal of Research in Medical Sci-
      ences* no. 18 (7) (2013): 573-579. https://www.ncbi.nlm.nih.gov/pmc/articles
      /PMC3897024/.

26   Koplay, Mustafa, Erim Gulcan, and Fuat Ozkan. "Association Between Serum
      Vitamin B_{12} Levels and the Degree of Steatosis in Patients With Nonalcoholic
      Fatty Liver Disease." *Journal of Investigative Medicine* 59, no. 7 (2011): 1137–
      40. doi:10.2310/jim.0b013e31822a29f5.

27   Medici, Valentina, and Charles H. Halsted. "Folate, Alcohol, and Liver
      Disease." *Molecular Nutrition & Food Research* 57, no. 4 (2012): 596–606.
      doi:10.1002/mnfr.201200077.

28   Tajiri, Kazuto. "Branched-chain Amino Acids in Liver Diseases." *World Journal
      of Gastroenterology* 19, no. 43 (2013): 7620. doi:10.3748/wjg.v19.i43.7620.

29   "DHA Study-Could Alzheimer's Be a Liver Disease?" ALZFORUM. http://
      www.alzforum.org/news/research-news/dha-study-could-alzheimers-be-liver
      -disease.

30   Deleve, Laurie, and Neil Kaplowitz. "Importance and Regulation of He-
      patic Glutathione." *Seminars in Liver Disease* 10, no. 04 (1990): 251–66.
      doi:10.1055/s-2008-1040481.

31   Bertot, Luis Calzadilla, and Leon Adams. "The Natural Course of Non-
      Alcoholic Fatty Liver Disease." *International Journal of Molecular Sciences* 17,
      no. 5 (2016): 774. doi:10.3390/ijms17050774.

32   Dyson, Jessica K., Quentin M. Anstee, and Stuart Mcpherson. "Non-alcoholic
      Fatty Liver Disease: A Practical Approach to Diagnosis and Staging." *Frontline
      Gastroenterology* 5, no. 3 (2013): 211–18. doi:10.1136/flgastro-2013-100403.

33   Brunt, Elizabeth M., Vincent W.-S. Wong, Valerio Nobili, Christopher P.
      Day, Silvia Sookoian, Jacquelyn J. Maher, Elisabetta Bugianesi, Claude B.
      Sirlin, Brent A. Neuschwander-Tetri, and Mary E. Rinella. "Nonalcoholic
      Fatty Liver Disease." *Nature News*, December 17, 2015. https://www.nature
      .com/articles/nrdp201580.

34   Caraceni, I. Grattagliano P., P. Portincasa, M. Domenicali, V.O. Palmieri, F.
      Trevisani, M. Bernardi, and Giuseppe Palasciano. "Adaptation of Subcellular
      Glutathione Detoxification System to Stress Conditions in Choline-Deficient
      Diet Induced Rat Fatty Liver." *Cell Biology and Toxicology* 19, no. 6 (2003):
      355–66. doi:10.1023/b:cbto.0000013341.73139.fc.

35   Spero, David, BSN, RN. "Healing Leaky Livers." *Diabetes Self-Management*.
      https://www.diabetesselfmanagement.com/blog/healing-leaky-livers/.

36   Kersten, Sander. "Mechanisms of Nutritional and Hormonal Regulation of
      Lipogenesis." *EMBO reports* 2, no. 4 (2001): 282–86. doi:10.1093/embo-reports
      /kve071.

37   Henkel, Elena, Mario Menschikowski, Carsta Koehler, Wolfgang Leon-
      hardt, and Markolf Hanefeld. "Impact of Glucagon Response on Postpran-
      dial Hyperglycemia in Men With Impaired Glucose Tolerance and Type
      2 Diabetes Mellitus." *Metabolism* 54, no. 9 (2005): 1168–73. doi:10.1016/j
      .metabol.2005.03.024.

CHAPTER THREE: HEAL YOUR LIVER

1   Hansel, Steven B., and Marilyn E. Morris. "Hepatic Conjugation/Deconju-
      gation Cycling Pathways. Computer Simulations Examining the Effect of
      Michaelis-Menten Parameters, Enzyme Distribution Patterns, and a Diffu-
      sional Barrier on Metabolite Disposition." *Journal of Pharmacokinetics and Bio-
      pharmaceutics* 24, no. 2 (1996): 219–43. doi:10.1007/bf02353490.

2   de Vries, E. M., L. A. Lammers, R. Achterbergh, H-J Klümpen, R. A. A.
      Mathot, A. Boelen, and J. A. Romijn. "Fasting-Induced Changes in Hepatic
      P450 Mediated Drug Metabolism Are Largely Independent of the Constitutive
      Androstane Receptor CAR." *Plos One* 11, no. 7 (2016). e0159552. doi:10.1371
      /journal.pone.0159552.

3   Hodges, Romilly E., and Deanna M. Minich. "Modulation of Metabolic
      Detoxification Pathways Using Foods and Food-Derived Components: A

Scientific Review with Clinical Application." *Journal of Nutrition and Metabolism* 2015 (2015): 1–23. doi:10.1155/2015/760689.

4   Navarro, S. L., J.-L. Chang, S. Peterson, C. Chen, I. B. King, Y. Schwarz, S. S. Li, L. Li, J. D. Potter, and J. W. Lampe. "Modulation of Human Serum Glutathione S-Transferase A1/2 Concentration by Cruciferous Vegetables in a Controlled Feeding Study Is Influenced by GSTM1 and GSTT1 Genotypes." *Cancer Epidemiology Biomarkers & Prevention* 18, no. 11 (2009): 2974–78. doi:10.1158/1055-9965.epi-09-0701.

5   Wark, P. A. "Habitual Consumption of Fruits and Vegetables: Associations With Human Rectal Glutathione S-Transferase." *Carcinogenesis* 25, no. 11 (2004): 2135–42. doi:10.1093/carcin/bgh238.

6   Lampe, Johanna W., Chu Chen, Sue Li, JoAnn Prunty, Margaret T. Grate, Diane E. Meehan, Karen V. Barale, Douglas A. Dightman, Ziding Feng, and John D. Potter. "Modulation of Human Glutathione S-Transferases by Botanically Defined Vegetable Diets." *Cancer Epidemiol Biomarkers* 9, no. 8 (2000): 787–93. http://cebp.aacrjournals.org/content/9/8/787.article-info.

7   USDA National Nutrient Database for Standard Reference. *Nutrient Data Laboratory. Release 27*. Washington, DC, Agriculture Research Service, 2011. http://ndb.nal.usda.gov/ndb/.

8   Reinke, Hans, and Gad Asher. "Circadian Clock Control of Liver Metabolic Functions." *Gastroenterology* 150, no. 3 (2016): 574–80. doi:10.1053/j.gastro.2015.11.043.

9   Yan, C. C., E. Bravo, and A. Cantafora. "Effect of Taurine Levels on Liver Lipid Metabolism: An In Vivo Study in the Rat." *Experimental Biology and Medicine* 202, no. 1 (1993): 88–96. doi:10.3181/00379727-202-43516.

10   Cameron, Meaghan. "Yes You Can...Lose Weight With Twinkies." *Reader's Digest*, May 23, 2016. https://www.rd.com/health/diet-weight-loss/yes-you-canlose-weight-with-twinkies/.

11   Campos-Nonato, Ismael, Lucia Hernandez, and Simon Barquera. "Effect of a High-Protein Diet versus Standard-Protein Diet on Weight Loss and Biomarkers of Metabolic Syndrome: A Randomized Clinical Trial." *Obesity Facts* 10, no. 3 (2017): 238–51. doi:10.1159/000471485.

12   Du, Yonggang, Ningbo Zhang, Meng Cui, Zhiqiang Liu, and Shuying Liu. "Studies of Interaction Between Insulin and Glutathione Using Electrospray Ionization Mass Spectrometry." *Rapid Communications in Mass Spectrometry* 26, no. 13 (2012): 1519–26. doi:10.1002/rcm.6248.

13   Iwen, K. Alexander, Erich Schröder, and Georg Brabant. "Thyroid Hormones and the Metabolic Syndrome." *European Thyroid Journal* 2, no. 2 (2013): 83–92. doi:10.1159/000351249.

14   Fernandez-Real, Jose-Manuel, Wifredo Ricart, and Roser Casamitjana. "Lower Cortisol Levels After Oral Glucose in Subjects With Insulin Resistance and Abdominal Obesity." *Clinical Endocrinology* 47, no. 5 (1997): 583–88. doi:10.1046/j.1365-2265.1997.3351120.x.

15   Pokusaeva, Karina, Gerald F. Fitzgerald, and Douwe Van Sinderen. "Carbohydrate Metabolism in Bifidobacteria." *Genes & Nutrition* 6, no. 3 (2011): 285–306. doi:10.1007/s12263-010-0206-6.

16   Abu-Elsaad, Nashwa M., and Wagdi Fawzi Elkashef. "Modified Citrus Pec-
      tin Stops Progression of Liver Fibrosis by Inhibiting Galectin-3 and Inducing
      Apoptosis Of Stellate Cells." *Canadian Journal of Physiology and Pharmacol-
      ogy* 94, no. 5 (2016): 554–62. doi:10.1139/cjpp-2015-0284.

17   Shen, Deqiang, Hao Bai, Zhaoping Li, Yue Yu, Huanhuan Zhang, and Liyong
      Chen. "Positive Effects of Resistant Starch Supplementation on Bowel Func-
      tion in Healthy Adults: A Systematic Review and Meta-Analysis of Random-
      ized Controlled Trials." *International Journal of Food Sciences and Nutrition* 68,
      no. 2 (2016): 149–57. doi:10.1080/09637486.2016.1226275.

18   Kieffer, D. A., B. D. Piccolo, M. L. Marco, E. B. Kim, M. L. Goodson,
      M. J. Keenan, T. N. Dunn, K. E. B. Knudsen, R. J. Martin, and S. H.
      Adams. "Mice Fed a High-Fat Diet Supplemented with Resistant Starch
      Display Marked Shifts in the Liver Metabolome Concurrent with Altered
      Gut Bacteria." *Journal of Nutrition* 146, no. 12 (2016): 2476–90. doi:10.3945/
      jn.116.238931.

19   Nöthlings, Ute, Matthias B. Schulze, Cornelia Weikert, Heiner Boeing,
      Yvonne T. Van Der Schouw, Christina Bamia, et al. "Intake of Vegetables, Le-
      gumes, and Fruit, and Risk for All-Cause, Cardiovascular, and Cancer Mor-
      tality in a European Diabetic Population." *Journal of Nutrition*, no. 138 (2008):
      775–81. http://jn.nutrition.org/content/138/4/775.full.pdf.

20   Alizadeh, Mohammad, Rassol Gharaaghaji, and Bahram Pourghassem Gar-
      gari. "The Effects of Legumes on Metabolic Features, Insulin Resistance and
      Hepatic Function Tests in Women with Central Obesity: A Randomized
      Controlled Trial." *International Journal of Preventive Medicine* 5, no. 6 (2014):
      710–20. https://www.ncbi.nlm.nih.gov/pubmed/25013690.

21   Tay, Jeannie, Natalie D. Luscombe-Marsh, Campbell H. Thompson, Manny
      Noakes, Jon D. Buckley, Gary A. Wittert, William S. Yancy, and Grant D.
      Brinkworth. "A Very Low-Carbohydrate, Low–Saturated Fat Diet for Type 2
      Diabetes Management: A Randomized Trial." *Diabetes Care* 37, no. 11 (2014):
      2909–18. doi:10.2337/dc14-0845.

22   "High Saturated Fat Diet in Teenage Years Raises Breast Cancer Risk Later."
      Nursing Standard 30, no. 41 (2016): 14. doi:10.7748/ns.30.41.14.s15.

23   Dumas, Julie A., Janice Y. Bunn, Joshua Nickerson, Karen I. Crain, David B.
      Ebenstein, Emily K. Tarleton, Jenna Makarewicz, Matthew E. Poynter, and
      Craig Lawrence Kien. "Dietary saturated fat and monounsaturated fat have
      reversible effects on brain function and the secretion of pro-inflammatory cyto-
      kines in young women." *Metabolism* 65, no. 10 (2016): 1582–88. doi:10.1016/j
      .metabol.2016.08.003.

24   Hodges, Romilly E., and Deanna M. Minich. "Modulation of Metabolic
      Detoxification Pathways Using Foods and Food-Derived Components: A Sci-
      entific Review with Clinical Application." *Journal of Nutrition and Metabolism*
      no. 2015 (2015): 1–23. doi:10.1155/2015/760689.

25   "Recommended Dietary Allowances." 1989. doi:10.17226/1349. https://www
      .nap.edu/catalog/1349/recommended-dietary-allowances-10th-edition

26   Piatti, P.M., L.D. Monti, Fulvio Magni, Isabella Fermo, L. Baruffaldi,
      R. Nasser, G. Santambrogio, M.C. Librenti, M. Galli-Kienle, A.E. Pontiroli,

and G. Pozza. "Hypocaloric High-Protein Diet Improves Glucose Oxidation and Spares Lean Body Mass: Comparison to Hypocaloric High-Carbohydrate Diet." *Metabolism* 43, no. 12 (1994): 1481–87. doi:10.1016 /0026-0495(94)90005-1.

27   Antonio, Jose, Corey A. Peacock, Anya Ellerbroek, Brandon Fromhoff, and Tobin Silver. "The Effects of Consuming a High Protein Diet (4.4 G/ Kg/D) on Body Composition In Resistance-Trained Individuals." *Journal of the International Society of Sports Nutrition* 11, no. 1 (2014): 19. doi:10.1186/1550-2783-11-19.

28   Raikos, Vassilios, Madalina Neacsu, Wendy Russell, and Garry Duthie. "Comparative Study of the Functional Properties of Lupin, Green Pea, Fava Bean, Hemp, and Buckwheat Flours as Affected by pH." *Food Science & Nutrition* 2, no. 6 (2014): 802–10. doi:10.1002/fsn3.143.

29   Mollard, Rebecca C., Bohdan L. Luhovyy, Christopher Smith, and G. Harvey Anderson. "Acute Effects of Pea Protein and Hull Fibre Alone and Combined on Blood Glucose, Appetite, and Food Intake in Healthy Young Men – A Randomized Crossover Trial." *Applied Physiology, Nutrition, and Metabolism* 39, no. 12 (2014): 1360–65. doi:10.1139/apnm-2014-0170.

30   Sirtori, Cesare R., Michela Triolo, Raffaella Bosisio, Alighiero Bondioli, Laura Calabresi, Viviana De Vergori, Monica Gomaraschi, Giuliana Mombelli, Franco Pazzucconi, Christian Zacherl, and Anna Arnoldi. "Hypocholesterolaemic Effects of Lupin Protein and Pea Protein/Fibre Combinations in Moderately Hypercholesterolaemic Individuals." *British Journal of Nutrition* 107, no. 08 (2011): 1176–183. doi:10.1017/s0007114511004120.

31   Beasley, Jeannette M., Marc J. Gunter, Andrea Z. Lacroix, Ross L. Prentice, Marian L. Neuhouser, Lesley F. Tinker, Mara Z. Vitolins, and Howard D. Strickler. "Associations of Serum Insulin-Like Growth Factor-I and Insulin-Like Growth Factor-Binding Protein 3 Levels With Biomarker-Calibrated Protein, Dairy Product and Milk Intake in the Womens Health Initiative." *British Journal of Nutrition* 111, no. 05 (2013): 847–53. doi:10.1017 /s000711451300319x.

32   Neacsu, M., C. Fyfe, G. Horgan, and A. M. Johnstone. "Appetite control and biomarkers of satiety with vegetarian (soy) and meat-based high-protein diets for weight loss in obese men: a randomized crossover trial." *American Journal of Clinical Nutrition* 100, no. 2 (2014): 548–58. doi:10.3945/ajcn.113.077503.

33   Weigle, David S., Patricia A. Breen, Colleen C. Matthys, Holly S. Callahan, Kaatje E. Meeuws, Verna R. Burden, and Jonathan Q Purnell. "A high-protein diet induces sustained reductions in appetite, ad libitum caloric intake, and body weight despite compensatory changes in diurnal plasma leptin and ghrelin concentrations." *American Journal of Clinical Nutrition* 82, no. 1 (July 2005): 41–48. Accessed December 16, 2017. http://ajcn.nutrition.org/content/82/1/41 .full.

34   Sutton, Elizabeth F., George A. Bray, Jeffrey H. Burton, Steven R. Smith, and Leanne M. Redman. "No evidence for metabolic adaptation in thermic effect of food by dietary protein." *Obesity* 24, no. 8 (2016): 1639–642. doi:10.1002 /oby.21541.

35   Johnston, Carol S., Carol S. Day, and Pamela D. Swan. "Postprandial Ther-
      mogenesis Is Increased 100% on a High-Protein, Low-Fat Diet versus a
      High-Carbohydrate, Low-Fat Diet in Healthy, Young Women." *Journal of the
      American College of Nutrition* 21, no. 1 (2002): 55–61. doi:10.1080/07315724
      .2002.10719194.

36   König, Daniel, Denise Zdzieblik, Peter Deibert, Aloys Berg, Albert Goll-
      hofer, and Martin Büchert. "Internal Fat and Cardiometabolic Risk Fac-
      tors Following a Meal-Replacement Regimen vs. Comprehensive Lifestyle
      Changes in Obese Subjects." *Nutrients* 7, no. 12 (2015): 9825–33. doi:10.3390
      /nu7125500.

37   Davis, Lisa M., Christopher Coleman, Jessica Kiel, Joni Rampolla, Tammy
      Hutchisen, Laura Ford, Wayne S. Andersen, and Andrea Hanlon-Mitola.
      "Efficacy of a Meal Replacement Diet Plan Compared to a Food-Based
      Diet Plan After a Period of Weight Loss and Weight Maintenance: A
      Randomized Controlled Trial." *Nutrition Journal* 9, no. 1 (2010). 11.
      doi:10.1186/1475-2891-9-11.

38   Gulati, Seema, Anoop Misra, Rajneesh Tiwari, Meenu Sharma, Ravindra M.
      Pandey, and Chander Prakash Yadav. "Effect of High-Protein Meal Replace-
      ment on Weight and Cardiometabolic Profile in Overweight/Obese Asian In-
      dians in North India." *British Journal of Nutrition* 117, no. 11 (2017): 1531–40.
      doi:10.1017/s0007114517001295.

39   Ibid.

40   Leader, Natasha J., Lynne Ryan, Lynda Molyneaux, and Dennis K. Yue. "How
      Best to Use Partial Meal Replacement in Managing Overweight or Obese
      Patients With Poorly Controlled Type 2 Diabetes." *Obesity* 21, no. 2 (2013):
      251–53. doi:10.1002/oby.20057.

41   Halton, Thomas L., and Frank B. Hu. "The Effects of High Protein Diets on
      Thermogenesis, Satiety and Weight Loss: A Critical Review." *Journal of the
      American College of Nutrition* 23, no. 5 (2004): 373–85. doi:10.1080/07315724
      .2004.10719381.

42   Verreijen, A. M., J. De Wilde, M. F. Engberink, S. Swinkels, S. Verlaan,
      and P. J. Weijs. "A High Whey Protein, Leucine Enriched Supplement Pre-
      serves Muscle Mass During Intentional Weight Loss in Obese Older Adults:
      A Double Blind Randomized Controlled Trial." *Clinical Nutrition* 32 (2013).
      S3 doi:10.1016/s0261-5614(13)60009-6.

43   "Sleep Loss Limits Fat Loss, Study Finds." *UChicago News*, May 17, 2016.
      https://news.uchicago.edu/article/2010/10/03/sleep-loss-limits-fat-loss-study
      -finds.

44   Kim, Seung-Jae, Hye Suk Kang, Jae-Ho Lee, Jae-Hyung Park, Chang Hwa
      Jung, Jae-Hoon Bae, Byung-Chul Oh, Dae-Kyu Song, Won-Ki Baek, and
      Seung-Soon Im. "Melatonin Ameliorates ER Stress-Mediated Hepatic Steato-
      sis Through Mir-23a in the Liver." *Biochemical and Biophysical Research Commu-
      nications* 458, no. 3 (2015): 462–69. doi:10.1016/j.bbrc.2015.01.117.

45   Hellmich, Nanci. "Sleep Lessens Effect of Genes on Weight." *USA Today*,
      April 30, 2012. https://usatoday30.usatoday.com/LIFE/usaedition/2012-05
      -01-Sleep-and-Kids-_ST_U.htm.

46   Heilbronn, Leonie K., Lilian De Jonge, Madlyn I. Frisard, James P. DeLany,
      D. Enette Larson Meyer, Jennifer Rood, Tuong Nguyen, et al. "Effect of
      6-Month Calorie Restriction on Biomarkers of Longevity, Metabolic Ad-
      aptation, and Oxidative Stress in Overweight Individuals: A Randomized
      Controlled Trial—Correction." *Jama* 295, no. 21 (2006): 2482. doi:10.1001/
      jama.295.21.2482.

47   Heilbronn, Leonie K., Lilian De Jonge, Madlyn I. Frisard, James P. DeLany,
      D. Enette Larson Meyer, Jennifer Rood, Tuong Nguyen, et al. "Effect of 6-mo.
      Calorie Restriction on Biomarkers of Longevity, Metabolic Adaptation and
      Oxidative Stress in Overweight Subjects." *JAMA:* 295, no. 13 (2006): 1539–48.
      https://www.ncbi.nlm.nih.gov/pmc/articles/PMC2692623/pdf/nihms105166
      .pdf.

48   Ashwell, M., P. Gunn, and S. Gibson. "Waist-to-Height Ratio Is a Better
      Screening Tool Than Waist Circumference and BMI for Adult Cardiometa-
      bolic Risk Factors: Systematic Review and Meta-Analysis." *Obesity Reviews* 13,
      no. 3 (2011): 275–86. doi:10.1111/j.1467-789x.2011.00952.x.

CHAPTER 4: PREPARE FOR A NEW METABOLISM

1   Ashwell, M., P. Gunn, and S. Gibson. "Waist-to-Height Ratio Is a Better
      Screening Tool Than Waist Circumference and BMI for Adult Cardiometa-
      bolic Risk Factors: Systematic Review and Meta-Analysis." *Obesity Reviews* 13,
      no. 3 (2011): 275–86. doi:10.1111/j.1467-789x.2011.00952.x.

2   Zeng, Qiang, Sheng-Yong Dong, Xiao-Nan Sun, Jing Xie, and Yi Cui. "Per-
      cent Body Fat Is a Better Predictor of Cardiovascular Risk Factors Than Body
      Mass Index." *Brazilian Journal of Medical and Biological Research* 45, no. 7
      (2012): 591–600. doi:10.1590/s0100-879x2012007500059.

3   Saxena, Arpit, Dawn Minton, Duck-Chul Lee, Xuemei Sui, Raja Fayad,
      Carl J. Lavie, and Steven N. Blair. "Protective Role of Resting Heart Rate on
      All-Cause and Cardiovascular Disease Mortality." *Mayo Clinic Proceedings* 88,
      no. 12 (2013): 1420x826. doi:10.1016/j.mayocp.2013.09.011.

CHAPTER FIVE: FOOD FOR THE METABOLISM RESET

1   Assy, Nimmer, Faris Nassar, and Maria Grosovski. "Monounsaturated Fat
      Enriched with Olive Oil in Non-alcoholic Fatty Liver Disease." *Olives and
      Olive Oil in Health and Disease Prevention*, no. 1 (2010): 1151–56. doi:10.1016/
      b978-0-12-374420-3.00126-1.

2   Ferramosca, Alessandra. "Modulation of Hepatic Steatosis by Dietary Fatty
      Acids." *World Journal of Gastroenterology* 20, no. 7 (2014): 1746. doi:10.3748/
      wjg.v20.i7.1746.

3   Barrera, Francisco. "Dietary Changes in Patients With Non-Alcoholic Fatty
      Liver Disease Are Independently Associated With Improvement in Liver

Function Tests." AASLD LiverLearning, (2012). https://liverlearning.aasld
.org/aasld/2012/thelivermeeting/24022/francisco.barrera.dietary.changes.in
.patients.with.non-alcoholic.fatty.liver.html

4   "Sleep, Exercise and Fitness: Is It Better to Sleep In Or Work Out?" *Time*
10/06/2015. http://time.com/3914773/exercise-sleep-fitness/?xid=time
_socialflow_twitter.

CHAPTER SIX: RESET LIFESTYLE

1   Kahan, V., M. l. Andersen, J. Tomimori, and S. Tufik. "Can Poor Sleep Affect Skin Integrity?" *Medical Hypotheses* 75, no. 6 (2010): 535–37. doi:10.1016/j
.mehy.2010.07.018.

2   "Radiometry and Photometry in Astronomy." Paul Schlyter 05/03/2017. http://
stjarnhimlen.se/comp/radfaq.html#10.

3   Qin, Tingting, Mulong Du, Haina Du, Yongqian Shu, Meilin Wang, and
Lingjun Zhu. "Folic Acid Supplements and Colorectal Cancer Risk: Meta-Analysis of Randomized Controlled Trials." *Scientific Reports* 5, no. 1 (2015).
12044. doi:10.1038/srep12044.

4   Joung, Ji Young, Yoon Young Cho, Sun-Mi Park, Tae Hun Kim, Na Kyung
Kim, Seo Young Sohn, Sun Wook Kim, and Jae Hoon Chung. "Effect of Iodine Restriction on Thyroid Function in Subclinical Hypothyroid Patients in
an Iodine-Replete Area: A Long Period Observation in a Large-Scale Cohort."
Thyroid 24, no. 9 (2014): 1361–68. doi:10.1089/thy.2014.0046.

5   Lewis, Joshua R., Simone Radavelli-Bagatini, Lars Rejnmark, Jian Sheng
Chen, Judy M. Simpson, Joan M. Lappe, Leif Mosekilde, Ross L. Prentice,
and Richard L. Prince. "The Effects of Calcium Supplementation on Verified Coronary Heart Disease Hospitalization and Death in Postmenopausal
Women: A Collaborative Meta-Analysis of Randomized Controlled Trials."
Journal of Bone and Mineral Research 30, no. 1 (2014): 165–75. doi:10.1002/
jbmr.2311.

6   Wu, Jian-Guo, Yong-Jun Kan, Yan-Bin Wu, Jun Yi, Ti-Qiang Chen, and Jin-Zhong Wu. "Hepatoprotective Effect of Ganoderma Triterpenoids Against
Oxidative Damage Induced Bytert-Butyl Hydroperoxide in Human Hepatic
Hepg2 Cells." *Pharmaceutical Biology* 54, no. 5 (2015): 919–29. doi:10.3109/138
80209.2015.1091481.

7   Ibid.

8   Winkler D. "Present and Historic Relevance of Yartsa Gunbu (Cordyceps Sinensis): An Ancient Myco-Medicinal in Tibet." *Fungi* 1 (2008): 6–7.

9   Jang, Min-Kyung, Yu-Ran Han, Jeong Nam, Chang Han, Byung Kim, Han-Sol Jeong, Ki-Tae Ha, and Myeong Jung. "Protective Effects of Alisma orientale Extract against Hepatic Steatosis via Inhibition of Endoplasmic Reticulum
Stress." *International Journal of Molecular Sciences* 16, no. 11 (2015): 26151–65.
doi:10.3390/ijms161125944.

10   Jang, Min-Kyung, Jeong Soo Nam, Ji Ha Kim, Ye-Rang Yun, Chang Woo
      Han, Byung Joo Kim, Han-Sol Jeong, Ki-Tae Ha, and Myeong Ho Jung.
      "Schisandra chinensis Extract Ameliorates Nonalcoholic Fatty Liver via In-
      hibition of Endoplasmic Reticulum Stress." *Journal of Ethnopharmacology* 185
      (2016): 96–104. doi:10.1016/j.jep.2016.03.021.

11   Xu, Xiaolin, Qian Li, Liewen Pang, Guoqian Huang, Jiechun Huang, Meng
      Shi, Xiaotian Sun, and Yiqing Wang. "Arctigenin promotes cholesterol ef-
      flux from THP-1 macrophages through PPAR-γ/LXR-α signaling pathway."
      Biochemical and Biophysical Research Communications 441, no. 2 (2013): 321–26.
      doi:10.1016/j.bbrc.2013.10.050.

12   Federico, Alessandro, Marcello Dallio, and Carmelina Loguercio. "Silymarin/
      Silybin and Chronic Liver Disease: A Marriage of Many Years." *Molecules* 22,
      no. 2 (2017): 191. doi:10.3390/molecules22020191.

13   Ibid.

14   Aller, R., O. Izaola, S. Gómez, C. Tafur, G. González, E. Berroa, N. Mora,
      J. M. González, and D. A. De Luis. "Effect of Silymarin Plus Vitamin E in
      Patients With Non-Alcoholic Fatty Liver Disease: A Randomized Clinical
      Pilot Study." *European Review of Medical Pharmacological Science* 19, no. 16
      (2015): 3118–24. http://www.europeanreview.org/article/9374.

CHAPTER NINE: MAINTENANCE

1   Monteiro, Carlos Augusto, Renata Bertazzi Levy, Rafael Moreira Claro,
      Inês Rugani Ribeiro De Castro, and Geoffrey Cannon. "A New Clas-
      sification of Foods Based on the Extent and Purpose of Their Process-
      ing." *Cadernos de Saúde Pública* 26, no. 11 (2010): 2039–49. doi:10.1590/
      s0102-311x2010001100005.

2   Holt, Susanne H. A., and Janette Brand Miller. "Increased Insulin Responses
      to Ingested Foods Are Associated With Lessened Satiety." *Appetite* 24, no. 1
      (1995): 43–54. doi:10.1016/s0195-6663(95)80005-0.

3   Lin, Lin, Hanja Allemekinders, Angela Dansby, Lisa Campbell, Shaunda
      Durance-Tod, Alvin Berger, and Peter J. Jones. "Evidence of Health Ben-
      efits of Canola Oil." *Nutrition Reviews* 71, no. 6 (2013): 370–85. doi:10.1111/
      nure.12033.

4   Knutsen, Helle Katrine, Jan Alexander, Lars Barregård, Margherita Big-
      nami, Beat Brüschweiler, Sandra Ceccatelli, Michael Dinovi, Lutz Edler, et
      al. "Erucic Acid in Feed and Food." *EFSA Journal* 14, no. 11 (2016). 173 pp.
      doi:10.2903/j.efsa.2016.4593.

5   Johnston, Bradley C., Steve Kanters, Kristofer Bandayrel, Ping Wu, Faysal
      Naji, Reed A. Siemieniuk, Geoff D. C. Ball, Jason W. Busse, Kristian Thor-
      lund, Gordon Guyatt, Jeroen P. Jansen, and Edward J. Mills. "Comparison
      of Weight Loss Among Named Diet Programs in Overweight and Obese
      Adults." *Jama* 312, no. 9 (2014): 923. doi:10.1001/jama.2014.10397.

6   Stockwell, Tim, Jinhui Zhao, Sapna Panwar, Audra Roemer, Timothy Naimi, and Tanya Chikritzhs. "Do 'Moderate' Drinkers Have Reduced Mortality Risk? A Systematic Review and Meta-Analysis of Alcohol Consumption and All-Cause Mortality." *Journal of Studies on Alcohol and Drugs* 77, no. 2 (2016): 185–98. doi:10.15288/jsad.2016.77.185.

7   "Get Moving to get Happier, Study Finds." *ScienceDaily*, 04/04/2018. https://www.sciencedaily.com/releases/2018/04/180404163635.htm.

CHAPTER TEN: FAQ

1   Brady, Carla W. "Liver Disease in Menopause." *World Journal of Gastroenterology* 21, no. 25 (2015): 7613. doi:10.3748/wjg.v21.i25.7613.

2   Bopp, Melanie J., Denise K. Houston, Leon Lenchik, Linda Easter, Stephen B. Kritchevsky, and Barbara J. Nicklas. "Lean Mass Loss Is Associated with Low Protein Intake during Dietary-Induced Weight Loss in Postmenopausal Women." *Journal of the American Dietetic Association* 108, no. 7 (2008): 1216–20. doi:10.1016/j.jada.2008.04.017.

3   Levin-Epstein, Amy. "Two Scoops of Quinoa." *Best Life*, October 2006, 66.

4   "The Benefits of Omega-3 Fatty Acids on Brain Health." *DrFuhrman.com*. 31/05/2016 https://www.drfuhrman.com/learn/library/articles/73/the-benefits-of-omega-3-fatty-acids-on-brain-health.

5   Mackey, John, Alona Pulde, and Matthew Lederman. *The Whole Foods Diet: The Lifesaving Plan for Health and Longevity*. New York: Grand Central Life & Style, 2017.

6   Cox, Christopher. "Consider the Oyster." *Slate*. 07/04/2010 http://www.slate.com/articles/life/food/2010/04/consider_the_oyster.html.

7   Klemmer, P., C. E. Grim, and F. C. Luft. "Who and What Drove Walter Kempner?: The Rice Diet Revisited." *Hypertension* 64, no. 4 (2014): 684–88. doi:10.1161/hypertensionaha.114.03946.

8   Kersten, Sander. "Mechanisms of Nutritional and Hormonal Regulation of Lipogenesis." *EMBO reports* 2, no. 4 (2001): 282–86. doi:10.1093/embo-reports/kve071.

9   Houten, Sander M., Sara Violante, Fatima V. Ventura, and Ronald J.A. Wanders. "The Biochemistry and Physiology of Mitochondrial Fatty Acid β-Oxidation and Its Genetic Disorders." *Annual Review of Physiology* 78, no. 1 (2016): 23–44. doi:10.1146/annurev-physiol-021115-105045.

10   Gan, Seng Khee, and Gerald F. Watts. "Is Adipose Tissue Lipolysis Always an Adaptive Response to Starvation?: Implications for Non-Alcoholic Fatty Liver Disease." *Clinical Science* 114, no. 8 (2008): 543–45. doi:10.1042/cs20070461.

11   Manninen, Anssi H. "Metabolic Effects of the Very-Low-Carbohydrate Diets: Misunderstood 'Villains' of Human Metabolism." *Journal of the International Society of Sports Nutrition* 1, no. 2 (2004): 7. doi:10.1186/1550-2783-1-2-7.

12   Hall, Kevin D., Thomas Bemis, Robert Brychta, Kong Y. Chen, Amber Cour-
      ville, Emma J. Crayner, Stephanie Goodwin, Juen Guo, Lilian Howard, et al.
      "Calorie for Calorie, Dietary Fat Restriction Results in More Body Fat Loss
      than Carbohydrate Restriction in People with Obesity." *Cell Metabolism* 22, no.
      3 (2015): 427–36. doi:10.1016/j.cmet.2015.07.021.

13   Hall, Kevin D., Kong Y. Chen, Juen Guo, Yan Y. Lam, Rudolph L. Leibel,
      Laurel Es Mayer, Marc L. Reitman, Michael Rosenbaum, Steven R. Smith,
      B. Timothy Walsh, and Eric Ravussin. "Energy Expenditure and Body
      Composition Changes After an Isocaloric Ketogenic Diet in Overweight and
      Obese Men." *American Journal of Clinical Nutrition* 104, no. 2 (2016): 324–33.
      doi:10.3945/ajcn.116.133561.

14   Díaz-Zavala, Rolando G., María F. Castro-Cantú, Mauro E. Valencia,
      Gerardo Álvarez-Hernández, Michelle M. Haby, and Julián Esparza-Romero.
      "Effect of the Holiday Season on Weight Gain: A Narrative Review." *Journal of
      Obesity* 2017 (2017): 1–13. doi:10.1155/2017/2085136.

15   Guérin, A., R. Mody, B. Fok, K. L. Lasch, Z. Zhou, E. Q. Wu, W. Zhou, and
      N. J. Talley. "Risk of Developing Colorectal Cancer and Benign Colorectal
      Neoplasm in Patients With Chronic Constipation." *Alimentary Pharmacology &
      Therapeutics* 40, no. 1 (2014): 83–92. doi:10.1111/apt.12789.

16   Bourassa, Megan W., Ishraq Alim, Scott J. Bultman, and Rajiv R. Ratan.
      "Butyrate, Neuroepigenetics and the Gut Microbiome: Can a High Fiber Diet
      Improve Brain Health?" *Neuroscience Letters* 625 (2016): 56–63. doi:10.1016/j
      .neulet.2016.02.009.

17   "Does Drinking Cold Water Burn More Calories Than Warm Water?"
      UAMSHealth, January 28, 2017. https://uamshealth.com/healthlibrary2
      /medicalmyths/doescoldwaterburnmorecalories/.

acknowledgments

I want to thank the following people for making this book possible. To my parents, Glen and Vivian Christianson, for giving me a love of learning and confidence in my ideas. To my other father, David Frawley, for inspiring me to write. To my children, Celestina and Ryan, for bringing me joy each day.

To the incredible team at Integrative Health: Sharon Anderson, Melinda Ashachik, Dr. Lauren Beardsley, Dr. Tara Burke, Mary Cinalli, Dr. Raquel Espinol, Jaime Gerber, Dr. Linda Khoshaba, Jamie Kurtz, Easton Lathion, Kim Lopata, Holly Penrod, Alex Perez, Dr. Rosalyn Ranon, Dr. Guillermo Ruiz, Josh Sorge, and Dr. Tiffany Turner.

Special thanks to JJ Virgin for showing me a greater vision of what was possible. To my literary team, led by Celeste Fine and Diana Baroni, for guiding the direction of the book and dialing in the details. To my favorite external brains, Dr. Guillermo Ruiz, Dr. Tiffany Turner, and Ari Whitten, who helped shape these ideas.

Thanks to the team that helped get this book out to the world, especially Amber Spears, Courtney Kenney, Brett Fairall, Laurie Balla, and Kirsten Womack.

Thanks to Michael Murray, ND, Paul Mittman, ND, and Michael Cronin, ND, for their roles in defining and expanding the naturopathic profession.

Final thanks to my lifelong hero, the late Dr. Carl Sagan, for his unparalleled passion and eloquence in sharing the grandest ideas.

ABOUT THE AUTHOR

Alan Christianson, NMD, author of the *New York Times* bestselling book *The Adrenal Reset Diet* and *The Thyroid Reset Diet,* is a naturopathic medical doctor who specializes in natural endocrinology with a focus on thyroid disorders. He founded Integrative Health, a physician group dedicated to helping people with thyroid disease and weight-loss resistance regain their health. He has been named a Top Doctor in *Phoenix* magazine and has appeared on national TV shows and in numerous print media. Dr. Christianson lives in Phoenix with his wife and their two children.

ALSO BY BESTSELLING AUTHOR
ALAN CHRISTIANSON, NMD

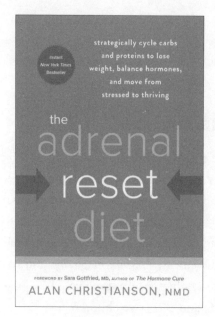

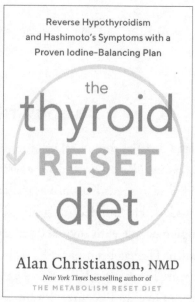

"All of Dr. Christianson's books are
required reading for my patients."

—SHAWN TASSONE, MD, PhD,
author of *The Hormone Balance Bible*

RODALE
BOOKS

Available wherever books are sold